For Youngae, with whom I've had so much fun discussing the quirks of being English.

And Hannah, for helping me discover a happy balance between my inner Margo and Barbara.

CONTENTS

countrymen and making a good impression.

Perhaps you are fascinated with the English, our lifestyle and the modus operandi of our supposed polite society (or at least what our charming media reports) and you are looking for ways to shoehorn some of that English gentility into your daily life. Perhaps you feel learning how to be a little more 'English' can help you get ahead of the game. I don't blame you, we English are known for our layers of charm and tradition which, until now, may have seemed like an alien nation with undecipherable social cyphers.

You have a longing to attend a traditional finishing school designed to create English lords and ladies, but have neither the ability to travel, nor pockets deep enough to attend one of the remaining few. Here's your opportunity. Though this book is modern and open to the masses, it still fiercely fights for the corner of tradition and 'doing things right', which is the very cornerstone of The Darling Academy's message—and England's, come to think of it.

Or simply, you are deeply driven by the wonderful chance to improve yourself every single day, and are interested in learning the nuances of living with other people, and how you can do this in the best way possible.

Regardless of your reason, I'm glad you are here. I bid you a warm welcome and offer you our congratulations. You are about to embark upon a guided tour of the principles for living your daily life like a refined, well mannered old time Englishman, or Englishwoman. I refrain from using the word 'typical' here, because truly good manners are sadly no longer typical of daily life. This is in fact a dying art and those who were raised with such class, moral obligation and understanding are a dying breed. We are drawing on the observation of a truly English lifestyle, one that is timeless, well mannered and well considered. Such lifestyles are either heavily romanticised or thought of as archaic to most people, yet we still adore the very idea of it nonetheless.

Historical and modern queens, princes, duchesses and counts, lords, ladies and debutantes are all raised and trained from birth under the watchful eye of parents, guardians, a nanny and governess who are there to correct and guide them on how to behave and what to say in all manner of social interactions. An extension to this education is the family. Each member well rounded, assured of the 'family brand' and sure of *position*. Every person surrounding a child is of *use* in educating him to become an upstanding citizen and one capable of passing on the family name.

The old time English who wished to embody this ideal countenance of grace and charm were known to embark upon personal improvement training within a residential finishing school. Happening upon or soon after a young lady's or gentleman's formal studies.,ladies of the middle and upper middle classes were sent to these finishing schools in order to train her for a lifestyle moving in elite circles and to establish herself as a good marriage option. For young gentlemen their training happened under the wing of mentors, uncles and fathers.

A mission and tradition that can, and should be carried forth today.

This may seem somewhat antiquated as an ideal, but the old English were shrewd and aware they were being observed with great scrutiny, they took every opportunity to 'level up' in the way they conducted themselves. An exercise much forgotten today, but to the few that do it, they cannot argue that it doesn't largely help you in business as well as achieving social success. The English who are confident in demonstrating good etiquette are widely thought of as those with 'good breeding', but for the purposes of equality and modern accessibility, we'll rephrase it to 'good training'. Good training can be sought by *all* who wish to pursue it.

Money and high position, networking, or a tight family unit used to be the only way to buy access to these principles and lessons but the modern world has changed and such information is now here for the taking. Regardless of your background you can now educate yourself on the principles of why your personal behaviour is of such importance and how to eliminate bad habits. Before you defend yourself, this isn't about changing who you are as a person, nor hiding from the past. Instead it's about smoothing those rough edges and giving you the confidence to be sociable with ease and grace from this day forward.

This is why I am absolutely delighted you have chosen to become PLU (people like us). No, not a snob, but a person *like us* who cares enough about *other* people to edit out unpleasantness for the benefit of those who surround you daily. You've been smart enough to save on the extortionate finishing school fees, and while you might not be rubbing shoulders with the great and good right now, learning a few inside tricks will certainly put you on the correct path to social and lifestyle success wherever you live.

This is not a book on how to be a snob, or dine with kings. Rather, a lifestyle guide on how to conduct yourself with grace, dignity and show respect to everyone you come into contact with. We are taking aged lessons and bringing them up to date to work in the here and now, while adding that little sparkle that sells British period dramas and detective series so well. Through this journey you will uncover not only the quirks that make the English who they are, but absorb yourself in a beautiful lifestyle choice that speaks of times past and shuns the frenetic unsatisfactory life to which most have become accustomed. Hooray for old time traditions!

This book will teach you to slow down, and how to do everyday things with grace.

If you are looking for etiquette diagrams of table settings and seating arrangements, you will not find them here. This information has been hashed out time and time again and it's of little use to duplicate. Besides, what use is that information in the average Joe or Joanna's day to day life? It certainly isn't relevant for most of us. Have you ever been exposed to or required the use of grape scissors or a snail tong? Thought not.

Instead, you will learn more about the *why* rather than an empty 'how'. Any great life lesson should begin with putting the heart and head in the right place before any steps are taken—theory before practical examination. Fret not, we shall cover that too so as not to leave you disappointed. My deepest honesty however; once you do learn the '*why*', the 'how' will often come about naturally.

Without further ado and mucking about in the school corridor, let's pull our socks up and get on with it shall we?

NOBILITY, GOOD STOCK & POLITE SOCIETY

A good life, well lived, depends on virtue

Noblesse Oblige: privilege entails responsibility

Well-bred, by definition doesn't mean you have to have been born into a well-heeled family or the aristocracy. If that were the case then only one percent of the British population would be considered well mannered. Frankly, that minuscule percentage sometimes does our great land a disservice because of their widely reported poor, and often embarrassing conduct.

The upper classes or "PLU" (people like us), a social inference coined by dear old novelist Nancy Mitford, are acutely aware of the old French term "noblesse oblige". Which simply conveys that those in a position of privilege are *obliged* to help those less fortunate. It denotes that nobility extends beyond a person's entitlements and requires that anyone who holds a status should fulfil their social responsibilities rather than live a self-interested life.

Can you say that about yourself and the people you know? Our world and the personal attitudes of the people living in it are changing beyond recognition, and sadly not for the better. Our modern cultures encourage very self-centred lives with 'to hell with it' attitudes. Little wonder then why our children are depressed, our marriages failing, and our debts increasing.

We have lost the meaning of what it means to be upstanding and a good example to those around us. We are no longer *noble* people.

Being noble means not only being generous financially where appropriate, but to be charitable with time, and most importantly **to be a beacon of good behaviour and proper moral conduct**. Just because someone might be born a lord or a lady doesn't mean they automatically are one. The circumstances to which you were born may give you a leg up the ladder or kick you down into the gutter, but by no means does it mean that you stay there by proxy.

Being of 'good stock' is to be well mannered and raised well enough to have been taught to always think of others before yourself. This is the very core of good etiquette.

Ideally we *should* be able to look to people in 'position' for pointers. This was easy to do in times past when the lord and lady who lived in the 'big house' were at the centre of our communities, but since rural life and their country gentlemen archetypes are a bit tired and passé, it would appear that we now *all* need reminders of the proper way to behave. The celebrities who grabbed headlines in times past *were* the aristocracy, forward a hundred years since the birth of television and social media, they are anything but. The only ones leading high profile lives and doing it *nearly* right are British royalty. Regardless of your personal tastes for monarchy, you cannot argue that they are well mannered, polite, socially aware and great diplomats. Of course, they are human like the rest of us and make mistakes, they are fallible and prone to slip ups but they remain acutely aware of *what really matters*. Which is, to *matter*. To matter to people, to matter for a cause. To live a life of purpose and meaning.

What really matters is being a good and moral person, leading by example and consistently trying your best.

It doesn't matter a jot about your genetics or family background. We are all able to learn and adopt the principles of noble living, no matter what our age or situation, and then work on improving them every single day of our lives.

A bank account with Coutts and an expansive country pile are not required for obtaining a genteel manner. Good manners are (and have always been) accessible to all.

The finest of English ladies and gentlemen are known to be masters of the following:

- Knowing 'what really matters'.
- Maintaining and being a good example of domestic harmony.
- Being level headed in conflict and measured in their emotions.
- Knowing the importance of being neat in appearance and practice good hygiene.
- To be well versed in the art of speech and conversation.
- Knowing that their opinions and needs are not greater than those of others.
- Being well versed in the rules of polite dining and public etiquette.
- Expecting and promoting high standards in all things.
- Surrounding themselves with life-giving language, pursuits and people.

You can always accredit these attributes to those of good stock, regardless of whether they have a healthy inheritance, a peerage title, or just barely get by.

Never forget that though you might not think you are in a leadership position or someone 'notable', your children and your peers *are* influenced by your actions and attitudes. Though you might not own a mansion, your modest home is *still* your castle. Though your marriage is not written about in gossip columns, the neighbour on the corner still notices your conduct. Perhaps you haven't made it to the position of director or shareholder yet, but you are *still* an influence to the office temp, your clients and your colleagues.

Every action you take, good or bad, influences someone, somewhere.

The world today is filled with so many messages about how to 'have it all', how to live a fast-paced aggressive life and often to the detriment of your heart, feelings and spirit. More often than not, what we are 'sold and told' today goes against everything that encompasses a refined lifestyle, good morals, strong personal boundaries and most importantly, the *enjoyment* of living according to those principles.

To realise that you are living life *now*, making the best of your position and your circumstances **on this very day** while *still* being able to conduct yourself politely and with decency and decorum is what it means to win at life.

It is possible to have a full and rewarding, joyful life *playing by the rules*. Your generation was not the first to discover what it means to have fun. Pre-sexual revolution life was full of social rules and obligations, but fun, family time, marriage, good friendships and social time still existed just as much then as it does now. You don't have to be badly behaved, act immorally or be self-destructive to feel like life is worth living.

Rule breaking gets you into more trouble than it's worth.

Just fifty years ago, lots of young men and women were taught good manners, standards and ideals as a matter of course. It mattered to people to uphold a good reputation and young adults actively wanted to know the ins-and-outs of doing it. Ladies were taken aside to be taught about feminine dignity, polite behaviour, personal conduct and how to behave in society *from a female perspective,* but now it is pretty much a free for all with 'celebrity' and trashy magazines telling us how to (mis)behave. Think about that. Aside from how to make a pie or combine an outfit, what did the last article you read concerning something to do with morals teach you? Was it clearly defining or did it leave you confused? Much of modern media cannot be trusted to teach you how to make good decisions, only selfish ones. 'Buy that', 'swallow this pill to get slim', 'sleep with a stranger tonight if you want to', then they'll tell you to do the total opposite in the next issue.

Previously our young men were taught how to treat women like ladies, and how to behave well in professional environments, usually by example from their fathers and grandfathers. Their mentors were a good example of a man's place and *worth* in a traditional family unit and had a good work ethic. Today, flashy footballers and boorish male TV stars are their only role models. While men have been encouraged to 'sow their oats', women have been told they don't need 'these men', so their sense of self-worth diminishes. The media opinion only backs this up, never celebrating the committed and loving husband and father of four, but instead promoting and encouraging the lad about town with the ready cash and gaggle of easy women on his arm.

Gone is the gentleman and along with him, the lady.

How many of our current contemporaries are teaching by example and providing a fine example for the next generation? It's hard to think of any, let alone count them.

Past social skills given to fledgling adults were both practical and personal; how to handle yourselves properly in society, what to do in awkward situations, how to present yourself pleasantly and what *not* to say was as crucial as what to say. It was a social narrative deemed important in the past. This may seem a little odd to us today, perhaps even a little contrived, but holding back on personal information, practicing decorum, propriety, constant politeness and dignity is not as easy for us today as it once was. This is because it isn't *expected* anymore. We live in a society where over-sharing of personal information is acceptable, and as such we get ourselves into all sorts of trouble, both with other people and to the detriment of our own self-confidence. We are always second-guessing our position in society, our identity, personal feelings and not knowing what is expected of us. Consequently our feelings of guilt, shame and social anxieties are amplified and our self-confidence plummets.

We take pride in our popularity, earning potential, sexuality, sexual and sporting prowess, rather than our kindness and compassion. Our young girls want to be glorified glamour models or reality stars rather than model wives and great mothers, because *apparently* that's what the boys all want in women. Men *apparently* want to conquer many women and treat them like sexual objects because that is the only thing which will demonstrate their ability to 'be a man'.

This is the very antithesis of English politeness. To be coarse and clumsy in your personal conduct and verbally boastful is the very *opposite* of what it means to have a good grasp on politeness and common decency.

We are becoming a self-obsessed generation with no regard for secrecy and decency. We compete with our neighbour rather than commune with them. We support our immediate family but not the community.

We must take a stand against the narrative that tells us that it's perfectly acceptable to be self-centred and live for our own pleasures. Humans were made for community, family and existing in an orderly, honest and supportive society. Isn't it about time we started living according to that truth?

Manners maketh man

Ask yourself why all English period dramas do so well. Is it because of the story? The history, the costumes? Or does it go deeper than that?

Mr Darcy is a romantic hero, but for a character with many faces (Colin Firth a favourite), are we in love with Fitzwilliam Darcy himself, or his conduct? Is the romance between Darcy and Miss Bennet really the key to our fascination or might it be the deep longing to live out a similar romantic exchange for ourselves? The ways in which they speak to one another so politely. How they hold back, the etiquette of courtship and the sweet sensation of allowing yourself to fall in love slowly rather than diving right in. The 'rules and manners', so plain to see, are the very essence of what endears us with their love story.

Of course, it's true there will always be characters through history that acted selfishly, broke hearts and wounded the feelings of others. They made it into the history books, infamous if you will, but they were never the popular ones. Lonely endings almost always befell those types of characters.

So who do you wish to be in the novel of your life? A romantic hero or heroine, greatly esteemed by all you meet? Or the curmudgeonly villain?

Any book written on the subject of etiquette cannot fix the problem of our society, or make every man and woman under the sun as nice as pie, but they can be used to great affect to make positive changes to your immediate circle and the *experiences* of your life going forward. It all starts with **you** as the central character to your life. You create your reality.

Where to start

Personal poise, elegance, self-worth, self-confidence, maturity and refinement is a never-ending *process* rather than a permanent state. Life is about constantly learning—no one ever truly 'arrives', and age doesn't make a blind bit of difference as we are all on a journey that does *not* end. Your spirit, or the *memory* of you will live on long after you are six feet under. So what path do you wish to take? What are you working towards, and are you doing it with dignity and grace?

What is the current state of your home and the person that resides there? What is the current state of *your heart and lifestyle* when you close the door on the world and stop pretending to keep up with everything? Do you like your habits, your surroundings, your interactions, your conduct and your lifestyle?

When you think about your life, are you enjoying it in a positive frame of mind?

Life runs smoothly when you stop fighting the world and instead choose to be polite *to* it. That means to your fellow man, and the earth itself. When you remain in a positive frame of mind and expect high standards from yourself and those around you, your work life, home and relationships run smoothly, not only from an operational point of view but for the sake of your sanity! It's no fun running around with a frown and griping at everyone.

In case we had all forgotten, politeness and domesticity are some of the highest ranking needs for survival of the soul. Maslow's hierarchy of needs ranked the following needs as greatest in all people, yourself included, in order of importance:

Self-Actualisation. The knowing of who you are, what your purpose is, and your identity. The need for personal fulfilment and *growth* as a person.

Esteem. What gives you self-esteem, helps you to achieve, *to have confidence, to be respected* and to learn *how to respect others.*

Love & Belonging. The need for *friendship*, love, and intimacy with others.

Safety. Your security, a roof over your head. A *sense of belonging* to a family, a *community where you share the same morals and principles*, to feel a part of something.

Physical needs. Warmth, comfort, shelter, food, and *feeling relaxed!*

In the world today we aren't encouraged to have much regard for the inward self, our relationships, or our community. It would appear we always need to be out seeking. Seeking more, seeking adventure, seeking 'stuff', yet think of your fondest childhood memories. Were they not centred around your home, around moments of *togetherness*, around those that you love? Can you remember how it made you *feel*? Was everyone smiling? Were you? Were things *simpler*? Perhaps if you aren't the keeper of memories such as these, don't you wish you had them?

Fond memories are made of good feeling, love, and acceptance and those are things that you cannot buy, but you can *create* them. Love, acceptance, forgiveness, belonging and feeling happy are not born from feelings of awkwardness, hatred, contempt and incivility.

You need to get your mind right about how you treat yourself and those around you in order to align yourself with good things and create a life to be proud of.

Good upstanding citizens are the powerhouse of any community. They are esteemed members of society, so why would you choose anything less for yourself?

The alternative is to be regarded as lazy, uninspiring, unmotivated, a drain on society rather than a cornerstone. Most people are a little bit lazy, or overworked, under appreciated, and bitter about it! This is because it is simply not fashionable or respected to want to learn vital etiquette and social skills anymore.

No one is standing up for the 'skill' of human to human social engagement, or moral obligation, or learning how to give sound advice and be an encouragement to others.

So what can we do about this lack of respect for ourselves as ladies and gentlemen and the traditional roles we wish to fulfil? How can we change the common opinion on the importance of politeness and help lift our cultural game?

All it takes is a little self-respect, being honest with yourself and a willingness to learn. When an individual takes pride in their identity and is truly confident in their ability to positively interact with others, they become some of the most influential and highly prized people in society.

These upstanding citizens are influencing and raising the next generation, as are their less-polite counterparts. Wouldn't you much rather know that a future employer, employee, teacher, friend, the spouse of your child, or indeed *your* future spouse was raised by someone with great manners and a respect for others and themselves? Rather that, than a self-centred, fame hungry and chaotic 'reality TV' type character? It sounds judgmental, but it *is* the measure of things right now.

Honour something greater than yourself

You can look to emulate the behaviour of current celebrities or negative influencers in your life who are consuming fast food, buying fast fashion, living mindless fast paced lives, chasing fast money—and in return live a negative, troublesome, dramatic life. Or look to great examples of considerate people who promote 'slow living'. There are many people that are choosing to walk a narrow path that goes against the grain of our modern culture, we call them 'old fashioned', and really quite 'quintessentially English'. On the surface, choosing to live a life full of old noble values might seem a little slow, boring or stifled, but 'polite kin' know the inherent truth that living this way is a kinder existence to the heart and soul.

Throughout this book we'll explore the depths of your heart and what will make you a master of etiquette, considerate living and personal refinement. We'll detail and explore the practical steps that will help you to embrace this lifestyle and how to make the very best of it. It doesn't matter whether you are a fresh-faced teen or decidedly long in the tooth, we all have *something* to learn.

This school requires no summer-long stays in a boarding house with a frightening headmistress, or balancing books on your head, but admission does require an open mind. It also deeply requires *admission* that you do not know everything and are willing to humble yourself in order to learn. Your ego and perception of your *own* self importance will be the greatest obstacle throughout this text and it *will* challenge you. This is a road less travelled, but it's a fantastic and beautiful journey. Embrace a life of noble kindness and keep good values at the centre of it, I dare you. It might just be the positive change you are looking for.

COMMON DECENCY IN ONE'S CASTLE

The Art of English Etiquette is Homegrown

Where the land is fertile, a good crop grows

You've heard it said that man's home is his castle. Whether you are a homeowner, renting, or still live with your parents, we all need to treat our home lives and the people we share a roof with a little better. In today's society I wonder if half the population really know the true meaning of the word 'home'. We are so used to moving from pillar to post, chasing the next best thing or up and coming postcode, we end up leaving behind all things safe and sincere.

A home is a place where one lives or has a presence permanently as a family member or collective household.

Since the sexual revolution of the 1960s there has been a steady move away from the social ideal which meant home was where your mother and father lived, along with any siblings. This was the bedrock of your family. It centred your identity, and your 'family' came as a whole. You were known by your surname, which went before you as an individual and it quite openly created a reputation, good or bad, that could follow you for life. You did all you could to respect and uphold your family name and playing by the 'rules' helped you to do that. Your address rarely, if ever changed more than once and home was a safe haven. Not many of us are lucky to have a typical, happy and harmonious nuclear family handed to us on a plate, but we should wake up to the fact that *we have the power to create it.*

Here in England we still crave these old-fashioned ideals and laud them as one of the things that make Britain great. We love our family nights in, listening to The Archers or watching our soaps and dramas that centre around family life (albeit with some rather far-fetched story lines). Our Royal Family are adored and our people still often plump for the 'traditional English church wedding or christening' in their home town or village, despite not being regular church members. The promise of a Sunday roast and the smell of mum's cooking makes us content. We like to know and trust our neighbours, we like to know the gent who runs the corner store and we get our curries and fish and chips from our tried and tested favourite takeaways. We are loyal to what we know, love and like. Our hearts beat with fondness at the sight of the same jolly lollipop lady who herded us safely across the road during our school years, or our favourite school dinner lady who now serves our own children.

There is comfort in familiarity and 'the done thing'. We really crave what is old and what is familiar. We crave the very idea of family and tradition, because these things are what make life stable and secure. *This* is what makes Britain great.

So what does this have to do with etiquette? Well, to play into the hand of an English lifestyle and demeanour you have to set your minds back three generations or so when family reputation really *did* matter.

Mr & Mrs Smith likely bought and moved into their house shortly after marrying and filled it accordingly with children. These children knew these four walls as their family nest and occasionally, or weekly, a visiting hoard of extra bodies in the shapes of aunts, uncles, cousins and much-adored grandparents appeared. Their home came alive with visiting friends and family life was centred around traditional routines and stability.

The Smith family knew and socialised with their neighbours, who also 'stayed put' in their homes. The youngsters played with the neighbours children in the street or in their back gardens. These children went to the local school and were known as the siblings of the older ones who had gone before. Neighbours also looked out for you, telling you off right then and there for being naughty if they caught you doing something wrong. The raising and monitoring of children was undertaken by the 'village'. Children respected their elders regardless of whether they were related, because it was instilled in them that this was *the way things are*. Social generational hierarchy and solidity meant that you were watched over by all adults in your community and you respected the rules of the street.

The family unit and the reputation they upheld (or didn't) were as real as the bricks and mortar of the home they lived in.

Now, it is very evident that this is *not* your typical family or social dynamic today, in most cases far from it. However, the appeal of this older family 'ideal' brings with it a solid purpose and greater meaning.

In almost any English street you will find one family who stay put. It is a rarity, but they can be found if you look hard enough. They know the area inside out and make their home their castle, no matter how modest it may be. Something you must do too if you wish to shoehorn a little old-fashioned English charm into your life, because the source of harmony, potential, good etiquette and a purpose for living lies right *inside* your front door. It lives in the heart of your own home.

Modern society has told us that the things 'worth' having are out there in the big wide world. The happy and fulfilling things in life are only found *outside* of home and have to be purchased. It leaves many in a perpetual tailspin chasing the next best thing or what sparkles the brightest. True English lifestyle and etiquette, and our grass-roots behaviour lies in *creating* a home to be proud of, a nest in which to rest. One that supports a strong family unit (however that may look), according to the good name we wish to preserve. This mission is central to creating and maintaining a unit of content, well-rounded individuals we support as a family and the children we are raising.

How you view and respect your home life and the family you share it with speaks volumes about your self-esteem, self-respect and how you wish the world could be.

You set the tone for your home.

English home management for a harmonious household

The old English are rather rigorous when it comes to the operation of their homes and the conduct within it. Surroundings and attitudes must always be ship shape. Respect for the home, familial decency, time honoured traditions and adhering to 'the done thing' is religiously upheld and expected. Some might think it all rather formal to look to these ideals, but in today's world the tables have turned with children now ruling the roost and 'modern' parents practically throwing discipline out of the window in favour of raising 'wild and free' children. These people are thinking short term. Charming little Maisie and Max are left to 'explore without boundaries', yet they see *not* the future annoying self-important, entitled 'darlings' they'll become in their late teens and early twenties. We've all met that type of child/teen/adult, the kind that are expecting life to happen *for* them rather than mucking in. We think them 'rude' (the parents *and* the children). Parents who adopt a chaotic and boundary-less form of home and child management are essentially making a rod for their own backs.

A return to English house rules is what's required if you want your home to run like a well oiled machine where everyone knows their place, pitches in, and no one person is put-upon. The only exception to the rules is the dog who gets free hugs and the leisurely life we all wish we had.

Father, mother, the children and the pets all know their place in the hierarchy of the English home and all play the role they have been assigned with a great sense of duty and pride. Ruling with an iron rod really does the world of good, but *only* when you back it up with a warm, loving and caring environment. Gentle, consistent, but firm is a world away from bullying, condemnation, and coldness.

Nurture a happy and loving household, but one that sticks by *the rules*. Live by them, be the example and expect the same from everyone. It really is that simple. New age parenting ideas are all well and good but we are aiming to create good characters and pillars of society, not spoiled superstars. Discipline and family expectations still have their place today when used for good cause.

Fastidiously and famously 'Family First'

You don't have to be a rocket scientist to know that families can be somewhat *interesting*, a little quirky, and at times downright dysfunctional. After all, you obtained association with these people by pure chance, not out of choice. What you must understand is that it is equally your effort towards common courtesy and understanding to make your unit work as it is theirs.

No family can stick together because of one singular person's efforts when the rest are pulling in different directions.

Admittedly it's nigh on impossible to teach old and disobedient dogs new tricks. If you are part of a family unit that behaves less than ideally, rather than reprimand them, shout, kick and scream, the best you can do, and what will get noticed, is to lead by example and hope that the rest of the family follow suit. If this doesn't make a difference then you can only look to the future. This is what the English are great at, dusting ourselves off, painting on that 'stiff upper lip' and leaving weak links behind.

You shouldn't live your life under the shadow of another person's embarrassing, antisocial and boorish behaviour. It is a cruel thing to gift yourself with a lifetime of feeling like a black sheep and mentally or verbally apologising to everyone on behalf of your family unit. Worse still to torment yourself with the misery of trying to fit in where you never will.

You can of course choose to have the patience of a saint, but be wise enough to know when to call it a day. It isn't polite to point out or correct another person's mistakes or etiquette errors when they have no desire to learn, nor should you have to put up with it.

Remember, what you allow to happen or be said in your presence says a lot about what you will tolerate and the standards you set for yourself.

If you are yet to have a family of your own, promise yourself that when you start a family in the future, the solidarity of that unit and its ability to thrive should be your utmost priority. If you already have your own family unit then by goodness, you must do this starting **right now**.

Societies thrive on strong family units, which contribute to strong communities that go on to build strong nations. In cities, the individual is there to earn money for himself, generally biding time until he finds a partner. In this environment you'll find crime rates are higher, poverty is prevalent, depression rates are higher and instability in both housing arrangements and business is rife. This is often because the *individual* is operating solo, with no one to consider but himself. He has become untied from the anchor and is adrift. Look to the suburban areas or where the majority of families live and you'll find things move at a slower, more determined and logical pace. Families provide a sense of belonging and a sense of pride in one's name and position in society. This not to say that suburban lifestyles are perfect, but family units that operate out of love and respect lift up and support a community as a whole.

Those who take the time to make sure their homes run beautifully and politely set a wonderful example to the outside world. Here's how your home and family can be a part of that movement.

Embrace the intimacy

Your home is a place in which to relax and feel safe from the outside world. The feeling should be palpable. Therefore it is of the utmost importance to establish and maintain a sense of serenity and calmness within your four walls. Insist that every family member, yourself included, has the decency to treat each other with respect and kindness. It is a sad fact that those we live with can cause our tempers to flare quicker than they would in the outside world. The close proximity of living with another humans' flaws, quirks and foibles is enough to ruffle the feathers of those with the steeliest nerves.

Learn to embrace the intimacy and quirks of those living with you and how to simply just let some things go. You might wish to suggest changes that might make living together more pleasant. You should expect your home companions to be keen to please the members of the nest, but relax and remember that not everything will run swimmingly all the time. Sometimes you have bigger fish to fry; a grumpy teen of a weekend morning, a husband who whistles too loud in the shower, or a dog that passes wind at inopportune moments might be irritating but you'd sure miss them if they weren't there.

Embrace the intimacy and the blessing of having people to live with and love, regardless of how much their habits might annoy. Question how the things that *you* do might annoy others.

Respect personal space

Whether you are named on title deeds for your property, renting a room or living with your parents, we all need to learn to respect the personal space of those we live with.

You should only ever enter a room with a closed door after knocking first; this rule doesn't just apply to lavatories, bathrooms or bedrooms! It applies to any room in the house that has a closed door; you never know what might be going on behind it. Some things may be pleasant (wrapping Christmas presents), and some things may be so shocking or graphic it will sear into your memory forever. Who wants to walk in and catch someone in the act of doing something they openly *chose* to hide from public view? Knock first, wait for a response and then enter. This rule applies regardless of your age or position in the family.

It is also good manners to ask if you can join a person who has already set up camp in a communal space. If they got there first, they have rights to use it as they wish. Do not automatically assume that because someone is in a shared room that you are welcome to fill the space and switch the activity to something that pleases you. Your father might like to watch the cricket on his own of an afternoon, or your mother might be enjoying a paperback in the sitting room, it could be the only time she has had to herself all day! Barging in and turning the radio on or making a loud phone call in the presence of people minding their own business is the height of rudeness.

The same goes for flatmates, their personal space is just as valuable as yours and you should do unto others as you would like done to you. If you set the standard of asking the simple question, "May I join you?", those who live with you will hopefully mirror this behaviour. It may seem formal but it shows respect towards the person you are asking and in the majority of cases the responses will be the same and you will be welcomed. If you get into this habit within the home, one day you might appreciate the open communication and ability to reply to that very question explaining that you *would* like some time alone. This is far more polite than huffing and stomping off to find solitude elsewhere.

Respect personal belongings

Those with siblings close in age will know all too well the frustration of not feeling as though you have things belonging solely to you. Though it is good manners to share, sometimes there are personal items and things within the home that an individual might cherish and therefore it is good manners to see that you respect the belongings of those you live with. This extends from something as seemingly insignificant as a hairbrush, through to books, clothing, and especially toiletries in a shared bathroom. Make sure to respect the belongings of others in your household, never use without asking, and demand that the same respect be treated to your things. Teach this concept early on with your children. The habit of thinking things can just be taken and used without asking is akin to stealing in later life. You may think a little blob here and there of your flatmate's shampoo or luxury hand cream isn't a big deal, but those help-yourself portions add up over time.

Do not interrupt

A rule to be keenly observed is the practice of not stealing conversation or attention. Interrupting someone in the flow of conversation or task is one of life's biggest annoyances and shows great disrespect. Allow someone to finish speaking, to wrap up their conversation on the phone or complete a task before you wade in and demand their attention. It is a good idea to teach young children that interruption is only acceptable strictly in an emergency, and they must wait for you to finish speaking before they can ask questions. Most likely an interruption is about something trivial anyway.

Another place to exercise this cardinal skill of patience is in shops and restaurants. I've lost count of the amount of people who have stolen a waiter's attention from right under my nose. It would serve the nation well for said waiters to refuse to turn their attention from me until we are done. If you are providing a service or having a conversation and find yourself being interrupted then recognise this as a way to *politely* remind people that patience is required if they desire your attention.

This simple sentence delivered in a kind and sincere tone is all that is required;

"Kindly hold on for one moment, let me finish up my conversation/task and then we can talk about it/I'll be right with you".

This statement works for any situation you find yourself in, both inside and outside of the home, and absolutely cannot be argued. Those that take offence expose their rudeness and impatience.

If you are at the receiving end of the interruption then sadly there is not much you can do. It is of little use to make a scene and publicly shame people. Use these situations as a reminder not to behave this way yourself.

Parenting Tip: Teach infant and primary age children that interruption is only acceptable in a true emergency (life, injury and hazardous situations, or lavatory emergencies only) and that they may demonstrate their need to talk to you otherwise by coming to place their hand softly on top of your hand, leg, or your forearm. They should stand still and quietly looking at you while they wait for you to finish. Use your spare hand and put it upon theirs as acknowledgment that you know they are waiting and are next in the queue to speak. Break your conversation at a convenient place, then turn your attention to the child. This works until they are old enough to understand the nuances of social politeness and have the patience to wait for your attention or a natural break in the conversation. Remember to praise them for waiting.

At an older age (pre-teens and up), teach them to precede their interruption into your flow of conversation with "Excuse me, but..." If what they say has anything to do with something *other* than the conversation they are interrupting, or an emergency, then they must seek to be excused for it. If they forget, never be afraid to gently but firmly correct and remind them of the proper way to interrupt you in front of company. The children will respond better to in-situation training rather than a strict telling off and screaming match behind closed doors once company has departed.

How many times have you been having an adult conversation with a spouse or friend and a child has interrupted to tell you something useless or trivial? Just because they are young does not make them more important. Claim back your right for adult respect!

Your hands are just as capable and your time is no more precious

A common affliction to those raised in a 'traditional' household whereby the wife and mother runs the home and takes on most of the household chores, is to think that she is there to serve you. Mothers and wives often like to take care of their husbands and offspring but *they must not* be taken for granted. If you take an attitude of expectancy and ingratitude, the person serving your meals and taking care of your laundry will eventually come to resent doing it. This only serves to breed an unharmonious atmosphere and feeling of contempt within the household. Make sure to *show* your appreciation, *speak* of your appreciation, and *offer* your help when appropriate.

If you are quite capable of doing something for yourself like making a sandwich, ironing a shirt, or even running a vacuum around the carpet, then for goodness sake do it! One way to show appreciation for the main caregiver is to gladly take on a task you don't mind doing. If you like vacuuming or weeding the garden and find it relaxing, then vow to do it, *without* having to be asked or expecting anything in return.

Be on time to dinner, and be well dressed

With those that serve you in mind, please be polite enough to turn up *on time* to the dinner table. Your mother/wife/spouse/flatmate has exerted a lot of time, effort and care in providing a meal for you (however simplistic), so do them the courtesy of being on time to the table. This does not mean arriving as the plate is put in front of you, but being there ready and waiting *before* your meal is served. You would do well to help take last minute items to the dining table or pouring drinks for others. This shows your appreciation and participation in the event, even if you haven't done the heavy stirring.

The home cooks who find themselves frustrated with waiting for those to arrive on time for dinner would do well to purchase a little brass bell to ring when the dish is five minutes from ready. Train your household to respond to this by finishing up their activities and making their way to the table. Hollering up the stairs for your children does not a respectful household make, and only adds stress to the meal when you are huffing and puffing that they haven't arrived at the table as you are dishing up.

Need it also be said that unless you are convalescing, pyjamas and states of undress are most inappropriate for the dinner table.

Remember to thank your provider for the meal and compliment the smell/look of the dish *before* you eat as well as showing gratitude after. Include details of what you liked about the meal to show that you paid attention. Be thankful.

No screens at the dinner table

It is one thing to expect your party to be on time to the table but they must also be *present*. The dining room is no place for the television and certainly not one for a mobile phone or tablet. The very point of sitting at a table is to execute the task of nourishing the body and forging intimacy with those you are dining with—this cannot be done in half measures. It is a great disappointment to see people eating and not paying attention and being grateful for the provision, taste and art of their food. Not to mention the lack of attention they give to those with whom they are sitting. Ban all screens at mealtimes in your home. It is better to sit in silence than endure the company of a dinner companion whose attention is elsewhere.

TV dinners are a personal choice, but make at least three a week an occasion to sit at the table. A shared weekend breakfast or brunch and a Sunday dinner should be the absolute minimum.

Pull your weight around the house

It goes without saying that all members of a household have a duty to help around the house. From the very young to the very old, there are tasks and chores that are suitable for all ages and abilities making for a very smooth operation if everyone knows what is expected of them. It is wholly unfair to leave all duties to one just person, even two, and children will eventually thank you for teaching them vital life skills no matter how much they protest at the time. Boarding school actually provides a great service in teaching young ones the demands of taking care of and the responsibility of oneself. Make these rules the **very least** your household members should each do daily:

- All beds to be made upon rising by the occupier, not a moment later.
- Dirty laundry must make its way to the designated area (not piled on the floor) ready for washing.
- All clean clothes must be put away by the wearer, not the washer.
- Dirty dishes and glasses to be put away in the dishwasher or rinsed and stacked neatly by the sink.
- Empty food containers to be recycled or thrown away.
- Shoes to be taken off upon entering the house and coats hung up.

As an aside, teenagers will likely be your worst protesters but by the age of twelve they must also be capable of and well practiced in:

- Operating a vacuum cleaner.
- Changing bedsheets.
- Replenishing bathroom consumables.
- Dividing laundry and operating a washing machine on a basic wash cycle.
- Correctly filling and emptying the dishwasher.
- Making a cup of tea.
- Buttering toast.
- Making a sandwich.

- Preparing a simple hot meal such as beans or fried egg on toast.
- Preparing vegetables.
- Obtain profound knowledge and awareness of personal and household hygiene.
- Taking out the rubbish and replacing bin bags.
- Going to the local shop and confidently buying items for the household from a basic list.
- Administering basic First Aid and responding calmly and efficiently in an emergency.

Having been raised in a household of many teenage siblings myself—most of whom went to boarding school—I can attest to the fact that though we doth protested at home and at school, we *were very* capable of mucking-in.

Don't let temper tantrums and laziness distract you.

If you don't want boomerang children that keep failing to launch, then it is your duty as a responsible parent to prepare your children for life's minor daily details as well as the bigger, more consuming ones. Trigonometry or which university to get sozzled at for four years means jot when your little cherub is incapable of making a decent breakfast or cleaning up after themselves. They will thank you in the long run, and you will thank yourself for raising capable humans to be proud of.

Once these tasks are mastered, feel free to leave them alone for a weekend. Only kidding. Kind of.

Keep the home clean

Though there are no rules for exactly *how* clean you should keep your home, there are some levels of decency to adhere to in order to operate a healthy, peaceful home. You might wonder how this sits in the subject of etiquette, but running a clean and delightful home *is* good manners. It affects the mental and physical state of all occupants and means that you are always ready to welcome guests into your house without grimacing at the embarrassing state of things. Remember, hygiene comes before orderliness, but maintaining a tight grip on both benefits the physical and mental state of your health.

This is an operation that requires communication and adherence by all parties in the home and you would do well to see the business of housekeeping as just that. Routines, delegation and expectation are the aim of the game here.

There are plenty of online resources to help you with the management of your home including daily task lists that will help you to keep on top of things. Leaving all jobs to one person on one day of the week is a surefire way to instil a hatred of housekeeping and make this essential part of your quality of life a bore, and a chore.

Plan out what you are able to tackle on what day of the week, and by whom, and stick to it. All parties should be able to make their beds, open curtains, put dirty clothes in the designated area and clean up breakfast things themselves. Even the youngest in the family are capable of this. Older children are able to dust, push a vacuum cleaner around the floor, and take out the rubbish. They are also quite capable of loading and emptying a dishwasher as well as putting away their own laundry. If they cannot do this, then for goodness sake, teach them!

For dirtier jobs, keeping anti-bacterial wipes in the bathroom is a quick way to clean up sink and toilet surfaces daily, making the weekly cleaning routine an overall lighter chore. Kitchen work surfaces should also be wiped down after every food preparation and put all dishes away ready for the dishwasher to be operated at night. This not only saves on energy, but keeps the surfaces free of clutter during the day. If you are without a dishwasher then wash up as you go. Leaving dishes and plates to fester all day on the kitchen work surface is not only unhygienic but makes for a depressing sight each time you enter the kitchen. If you must leave them to do all at once, rinse them first and stack neatly to tackle at the designated time.

It goes without saying, that the most important parts of your home to keep scrupulously clean are the kitchen and the bathroom. The preparation of food requires a sanitary workspace and I need not mention why the bathroom needs particular attention.

Not all Englishmen are house-proud, and to be honest, many err on the side of a little messy and rough round the edges than show-home status, but cleanliness and hygiene are a requirement for decent living. A little dog hair on the sofa, or dust on the mantle can be overlooked if the bathroom is of suitable condition and the food you serve guests came from a clean kitchen on spotless dishes.

If you find it hard to keep on top of your housekeeping then do make it easier on yourself by reducing clutter. The less you have lying around, the less there is to clean and dust.

Remember to say please and thank you

To have to include this pointer at all is rather sad. We all prick our ears at the great gaping void where a "Please" or "Thank you" should have been. We notice it acutely in strangers all the time, but one of the areas you *must* be strict on is the use of please and thank you within the home. It is so easy to fall into the trap of dropping your Ps&Qs when asking for things from your spouse, flatmates, and relatives, but this is the beginning of a downward spiral in manners and common courtesy. Children especially, learn by example. They are also not exempt from receiving *your* politeness.

What you allow to happen inside the home in terms of manners and decency will eventually creep into your daily lives outside. Remember that what you practice in the quiet of your own home is evidenced in the street—good and bad. Magic words cost nothing and they certainly make relationships richer.

Good morning, goodbye, and good night

Greeting people is one of the easiest ways to brighten the day. Acknowledging another person's existence and presence costs nothing but brings a richness that cannot be purchased. Have you ever noticed how the older generation are more likely to greet strangers in the street? A simple "Good morning", "Good day", or "Good evening" is all it takes to make you feel valued and part of society. It makes you feel *seen*. This is no different inside your own four walls.

Make it a rule to greet all members of your household good morning, wish them well when they leave the house, say hello when they return, and bid them a goodnight at the end of the day.

Feeling valued and seen in a household is a sure way to make all members feel part of a team. In our household it is considered a sin to not greet a family member in the morning or bid them goodnight. It keeps everyone accountable to one another and communication channels open. If you make allowances and excuses for ignoring each other in the house, what else can or will be ignored?

Community Tip: Greeting people on the street can also make things safer for you and your family, as well as the wider community. When you look people directly in the eye, you acknowledge their existence, put yourself in their frame, and is akin to saying, "I'm here, and I see *you*". Your community are much more likely to look out for you when they begin to recognise you. It is also a good way to avoid any potential threats from unsavoury characters. If you look them in the eye and really **see** them, they are less likely to consider you a potential victim. Keep your head high, your eyes open, your ears free from headphones, and your mouth ready to speak.

Brighten someone's day

Quite often, we are under the false assumption that we are here on Earth to enjoy ourselves as much as possible and look out for our own best interests. Yet, if you want to have a normal and healthy relationship with a partner, spouse or child, you might have to do something *for* someone else from time to time without expecting a single thing in return. This is easier with children, but easier said than done when it comes to adults. You may have to *care* about how a significant other is feeling, and actually *do* something about it. Wait not for when they hit rock bottom and scream out for help, instead do things to brighten someone *else's* day. Even little things like making a cup of tea and bringing it to your spouse or parents in bed, unloading the dishwasher without being asked, or getting the vacuum cleaner out when you notice the floor needs cleaning. You could even go so far as to buy a bunch of flowers, they needn't be expensive, or a small treat like a chocolate bar to bring home for everyone in the house. Open your eyes to your family unit being a big ball of collective energy and aim to keep it vibrating at a happy level. Everyone deserves care and attention. If your wallet is bare, don't forget that kind words cost nothing. Paying a complement or having a cheery conversation may be all it takes.

If you aren't part of an immediate family unit just yet then apply this method to those you spend most of your time with. Colleagues, friends, clients… What can you do to make someone's day a little nicer?

Respect quite times in the house

In order for your household to be peaceful and harmonious, there must, at times, be peace. This includes no loud music, loud television, shouting or making a scene. With children about this is hard to police, but making a point of having weekly quiet time and creating a culture from it could bring you the results you seek. Sunday is our day of rest, which means all activities are generally quiet ones from the moment we wake to the time we go to sleep. Of course, we do things as a family such as watching movies or playing board games and sharing a lovely family meal where chatter and laughter abounds but the emphasis is on low volume and togetherness. Though it may get noisy at times, it is the sound of togetherness and isn't coming at you from different areas of the house. This means switching off any devices, not allowing the communal areas to be given over to singular activities (football highlights on the television, dance practice from pre-teens or boisterous play for little ones) and instead focusing on activities where everyone is involved. It creates a feeling of calm and quiet even though there may still be a little noise.

It is also useful to instil a daily 'noise pollution' rule after a suitable time in the evening, say 8pm which *everyone* must abide by. Television and music volume must be reduced, or cut off completely and 'indoor voices' must be used by all. Should children remain awake past curfew, they must be quiet like mice, recognising it as 'adult time'. During adult time, priority is on quietness and adult conversation. This serves well for the peace of the household and your neighbours too. Not only that, you might find bedtime routines easier, calmer and less fuss made as children will find this time of day *boring*. Call it a win-win situation, calmer evenings and peace for all involved.

No shouting, raised voices, or slamming of doors

As the world's inhabitants transition into an impatient sort, it would do you well to remember that your feelings aren't always at the top of the tree. There are eight billion people in this world and what may anger you might not matter a jot to your neighbours. It's poor manners to expect them to be pulled into your arguments through the walls. Your raised voice and slamming of doors will only be met with equal aggression from your family, so is it really worth having a prickly temperament?

We all get frustrated and angry at times, but 'fighting fire with fire' never works. You must turn your attention instead to working on controlling your temper and diffusing a situation as soon as possible. In general, when things get heated women like to talk things over and men like to retreat into their caves, so you can see how much of a bind we can find ourselves in. This is normal. What isn't normal is the desire to explode with every fibre of our being in order to hurt the other person or prove them wrong. The English learn how to contain this primitive reflex and instead choose to deal with any conflict, quietly. We also don't always need to be right, but we do need to get along. Raising voices, slamming things and damaging your home is not good manners and will only serve you with regret once things have simmered down.

To maintain your cool when things get heated in your home, do any of these things to instantly restore a feeling of calm:

- *Choose* to finish your argument quietly and calmly, *it doesn't have to finish how it began.*
- Apologise for the situation you are in (the fact that you are fighting) Note: this is different from an apology. Express how sorry you are that there is

conflict and that instead you would like to talk about this peacefully.

- Go for a walk or pick up a menial task to allow yourself to calm down. Scrub the bathroom or go for a run! Burn it off in a positive, productive way.
- Stay away from alcohol, it only serves to amplify and sway your feelings and opinions—and they *may* not be the right ones.
- Allow your sparring partner to retreat to their cave if they need to. It may be a spouse, flatmate, or child but we all need space to 'decompress' sometimes. We can get so worked up we can't see the wood for the trees and when you allow people the space to retreat, they often emerge less tempered and able to see things from your point of view.
- Realise that nothing is ever the end of the world. Despite how you were wronged, the sun will still rise again tomorrow and you have the power to elevate yourself above *any* circumstance or negative situation.

It is well documented that the English like to 'put on a stiff upper lip' about things. To expressive Americans and more 'passionate' nations this seems like a rather rigid and less liberating way of living and dealing with our emotions, but I'd like to offer you an alternative view. Rather than looking at the stiff upper lip as a flaw, instead see its strength. How many times have you found yourself embroiled in an argument or heated situation that has nothing to do with you? Or found yourself an unwitting and unwilling counsellor to some stranger who airs their dirty laundry to anyone who will listen?

The English realise that their messes are their own to deal with and do so as quietly as possible. This does not translate as an excuse not to get help and support where needed, but does Mary next door *really* need to hear you arguing about who last took the bins out? Or does your colleague really need to see you moping about because you split up with your latest love interest? Sometimes you need to pull your socks up, keep calm and carry on. Everything blows over in the end and you should learn to refrain from fanning the flames where possible.

In addition, an address to husbands and wives: Petty arguments and passionate fights should never be witnessed by your children and the opinions of your children should certainly never be sought out for validation of who is right. The same should be said for bitterness and awkward silences. You are old enough to bear children, you should be mature enough to not let your mood sour your family atmosphere. You are part of a leadership team and despite what conflict you might find yourself in, you should never share your gripes with your subordinates. It isn't fair to lump adult issues on the children, no matter how grown they may be. It undermines the relationship between you and your partner. Let no child see the chinks in the armour of your marriage. Deal with your relationship in private because doing so publicly causes anxiety and a sense of unease in the children, which is wholly unfair. What may seem like a silly little argument to you and your spouse, may have rocked the foundation of the trust your children have in your partnership and can shape expectations for their own in the future. Respect their need for stability as much as your own.

Share everything and nothing

Speaking of sharing what goes on behind closed doors, there are some things you should share and a lot of things you shouldn't.

The sharing of private family information and gossip is beyond inappropriate. Never share the following information with those outside your immediate family unit:

- Financial information including how much you or your partner, or your parents earn.
- Details of addictions, arguments, personal dislikes and shortcomings of your spouse.
- Private career details and strategy belonging to your spouse.
- How much you (may) dislike your in-laws or your spouses extended family members.
- Sensitive medical information that is not belonging to you.

There should be a clear set of boundaries within your family of what is and isn't discussed with those that do not share your surname. Be disapproving of any conversation that looks like it is taking a sharp turn into these sensitive waters. Change the subject immediately. Expect your spouse, partner and children to keep family information to themselves and most importantly, explain why.

Why? Because things can change on a sixpence and what you overshare can soon become gossip and ammunition that can be used against you, whether you expect it or not. It can also be yesterday's news that people can hang on to. You will never truly know the agenda of others so the closer you keep your cards to your chest regarding your family the better. If your neighbour knows what you earn or how much you are in debt then any new purchase or financial decision you make will be met with judgment. If your husband or wife is having a rocky time at work, hates their boss, or things are frayed with a family member, then loose lips and what is said about the situation can often make its way to the wrong ears. What goes on behind closed doors should remain there. If you need help or professional opinion, then seek it out. Never expect your neighbour or best friend to know what to do. They may be a great sounding board, but gossip achieves nothing. By all means lighten the load and speak about things sensitively to the right ears if you need to, but realise that they are not there to fix your problems and may have an opinion or opposing point of view on the situation that could upset you. Be prepared for that.

Listen to and obey the head of the house

Like it or not, there is a head of your household. Though marriage is most definitely a partnership, despite this equal but very varied set of responsibilities, there will always be one top dog. If it pains you to admit it, just ask yourself who is really the one who handles things in a crisis? Who will pick up the pieces and support the family unit if the proverbial hits the fan? Who would you look to to defend your home and babies with all their might from an oncoming social collapse or apocalypse?

Traditional English households conform to the dynamic of having the father as the head of the household. He is responsible for supporting, providing for and protecting the family unit with his wife in full support of him, taking care of the smaller and often nicer details around the home. Whomsoever pays the majority of the bills and supports the family in strength and defence *is* the head. This does not give them free rein to abuse their position, but they should absolutely be respected. Heads, after all, are the last port of call in emergencies and the ones who have to put themselves in the firing line. The position of head really isn't to be envied as they have a lot of weight and responsibility on their shoulders and as such should be respected and treasured.

When the head and his support come together to create house rules, then these should be heeded. Be it financial restrictions, what behaviour is not acceptable under his roof, and the family rules everyone is expected to live by. Expectations may be high, but frankly, the person in the highest position should be lauded. Just as you would do as your employer asks of you in the workplace, so should be done in the home. This respect is **only** deserved by heads who run their ships with decency, fairness and love. Wives, do not resent your husband if he is in this position, but instead look to support him in his decisions. A marriage is a meeting of minds, but if you find that the CEO of your home is running you into rocky waters then you should speak up. Remind yourself also that where there is great responsibility, there is also great stress. Act kindly towards the head of your house and speak words of encouragement, kindness and thanks to them regularly for all they do.

The same will be returned to you. To not be the head of the house does not strictly mean to be 'put upon' by proxy.

Children should know that the mother and father come as a unit, but the head of the house has the final say. It is useful sometimes for a parent to refer to the head of the home to back up their position of authority. It is not a case of being under minded but instead *affirmed* in the eyes of the children. If they know that mother/father always agrees with the other and there is no argument in the matter, they'll do as they are told by either parent.

When everyone knows their position and identity in the family, such as head, support or underling, then families can be free to get along and express the nuances of their identity. If there is confusion in the ranks of who to listen to and obey then no wonder the kids run riot and warring partners argue.

In order to have a successful home you must run it like a tight ship, because ships can't sail far without a captain.

Your spouse comes first

"What has been joined together, let no man put asunder". This timeless statement regarding the sanctity of marriage does not only apply to those outside your four walls, but to all whom reside inside them. It doesn't only apply to those who consider themselves religious either. As a cohabiting newly married couple it is seemingly effortless to put your spouse first at home, but when little ones come along the attention you give your spouse often diminishes and the romance sadly wanes. You must do *everything* in your power to make your spouse feel of importance in your home. They are—in most cases—the reason you have a home in the first place. A house without family is simply a dwelling place. A house with family is a home, so do not let new additions to the fold slowly tear the very foundation of your union apart.

Parents and partners come first, end of story.

Think of the matter of your household and the family within it like a business, like a brand. Everyone must know their place, and like joint CEO's you and your spouse must ensure the fine running of the operation. You must ensure that all underlings are toeing the line, pulling their weight and upholding the values of your family. You must expect them to obey the rules that your coalition has put in place. Like good business partnerships, marriages rely on communication and shared time. Do not promote the importance of your teenager or child above your spouse, you cannot run a household in partnership with all attention on those less qualified.

Make time for one another and ensure that the family are aware that this is *necessary* for marriages and partnerships to survive and thrive.

Rules for good partnerships at home are:

- All decisions made by the partnership are final, and not to be undermined by subordinates. These rules stay in place even if one partner is out of the picture temporarily.
- Children must be respectful to *both* parents and not try to win one over in order to change the opinion of the other.
- Parents must demonstrate respect for their partner in front of their children. There is to be no badmouthing or complaining about their spouse in front of them.
- Parents must ensure that they have sufficient 'sacred time'. This means a set time in which children must be in bed so the parents can relax alone. Children are not permitted in the bedroom of the parents, or for cuddles on the sofa during this time.
- Allow the love for your partner to be *seen* in front of the children. Kiss, compliment and communicate. **You** are the models for your children's future relationships. Set a good example.

Show respect to your elders

A reminder for grown adults: You are never too old yourself to remember that respect towards the older generations is a *requirement*. This covers your parents, aunts, grandparents and older people in the community. A few decades ago this was an easier pill to swallow, since many of our older peers went to war to fight for our freedom—it was easy to see what they sacrificed for us. Yet, we must not let our ability to respect our elders be based solely upon what they do or have done for us.

Spending your days reading inspirational quotes from those older and wiser is of no use if you cannot tip your hat to your ageing neighbour. They may be just as wise as those whose advice you seek from yesteryear.

They were once part of a generation that 'ruled'.

Our older generations are often wiser and have a wealth of knowledge that is just waiting to be uncovered. Never think that an elder is 'past it' and cannot identify with your problem or current situation. This is narcissism and entitlement, to think that your modern opinion and ways of doing things is best. One day soon you too will have to give up your golden crown to the younger generation that are biting at your heels, just as your elders have done for you.

Community Tip: Honouring the following rules is a great way to teach your children how to respect their elders:

Give up your seat. Not just on public transport, but in public waiting rooms and private residences also. As willing as you are to give up your seat, you must not insist if they choose to decline your offer. Older people should never be made to feel like they no longer have free will over whether or where they seat themselves, just because someone was polite enough to give up comfort for them.

Listen and acknowledge. Lots of older people are genuinely lonely, and others just like to chat. If you really aren't in a hurry (be honest with yourself about how busy you really are), then stop and have a chat if an older person wishes to speak with you. I have had many fascinating conversations with people in unlikely places, and the stories they tell me are often so wonderful it makes it hard to tear myself away! Give your time and your attention. Restricting your only conversations to those the same age as you can, ironically, get old! Expand your horizons and be willing to talk to any generation. You might learn something new, and make a new friend.

Remember them. Easier said than done, but connect with the older generation living within your community and make sure to assist them if and when needed. When it snows and you are heading to the shops, call in on them and ask if they'd like you to pick up something for them. Invite them over for a cup of tea or a lunch on occasion. Send your older children over to mow their lawn or help with garden work.

Love your children but don't adore them

We live in a modern culture that is geared towards the over indulgence of our children and their entertainment than ever before. Where once children were allowed to play in the street, get into scrapes, and encouraged to make their own entertainment, we now wrap them in cottonwool and fill their diaries with expensive activities that drain our bank balances as well as our energy. It is crucial to engage with your children and make them feel important but it is another thing entirely to make them the centre of your universe.

Parental love is one of the most powerful forces on Earth, but if you want to raise polite, well rounded and grounded children then it would do you all well to help them to realise that life is not all about them. More importantly, that their entertainment sometimes has to come from their own imaginations and not always spoon-fed to them by adults.

The aim is to balance the old attitude of 'children should be seen and not heard', with the modern opinion that 'children are the most important thing in our lives, to the sacrifice of ourselves'.

It is *vitally* important to love and nurture your children, aiming to raise them in a happy and stable environment. However, they must be very aware during their formative years that the family is there as a unit, which they are a part of, but it does not exist *because* of them. This change in dynamic means many positive things for the family as a whole and for the child individually. Namely, learning how to respect people of all ages within the family unit. It is of no use spending all your time making sure your children are contented little piglets when your marriage is suffering, your spouse feels ignored, or you yourself are utterly drained of any time for your own nourishment, both physical and spiritual.

Raising your children under a blanket of love, but not adoration, will help them to realise that other people's feeling matter and that healthy relationship dynamics mean that everyone's feelings and comfort are important. It is good manners to realise that the world keeps turning with you in it, not because of you.

Self-centred attitudes are never attractive, so don't leave it too late to teach your children this humble lesson. Love them, but do not worship them.

Set your household boundaries

The advice on the etiquette of boundaries here is twofold; Firstly, your own personal boundaries, and secondly the boundaries your household in its entirety fall under.

Personal boundaries are the rules in which you intend to live by yourself and what you deem acceptable to you when cohabiting with other people. This includes with your children and spouse. For instance, you may impose a boundary that children are not permitted to enter your bedroom unless invited. This may seem a little stiff, but as a parent this room is potentially your only sacred space in the whole house. When those children are grown, how can they expect you to respect *their* personal bedroom space if they never had respect for yours? In our household, our son is often invited into our bedroom for morning cuddles, but he is not permitted to enter unless myself or my husband are in the room and allow him in. This is not something that we have told him he mustn't do, but on the couple of occasions he has been found to be in our room, we ask him to step out and say that he is not to be in there if we are not. The teaching here is that he isn't 'naughty' for going in, but it is just something 'we do not do'.

Another imposed boundary is that the upper level of our house is for rest and relaxation only. That means unless it is night, or you have gone upstairs to complete a task, you are not to be up there. Only books are permitted in the bedroom, no toys or screens. Not only does this keep our sleeping quarters quiet and peaceful, it means that we are together a lot more as a family in our living space. Children's bedtimes are also less of a battle with fewer distractions to contend with.

Boundary rules for children are also helpful with home office workspace, hazardous places like garages and work sheds and also cupboards where chemicals and medicines are kept. A stern word and constant reminders are all that are required to enforce the rules. It doesn't pay to shout and scream at your children in order to get your point across, a firm tone and a justification as to *why* they aren't permitted is enough. Should your children consistently disregard these rules, then it's time to communicate to them the consequences for their disobedience.

With regard to living in a household with peers, it is definitely not right to reprimand or give everyone a telling off, but instead to live by example. Do not enter spaces that do not belong to you and demand the same level of respect in turn.

Have respect for the household kitty

Effectively managing your personal finances are a bittersweet fact of life. Great when things go well, but a sorry story when the chips are down. It is important for your family's wellbeing to remain consistent in your spending so that you never live beyond your means. Many families and marriages are torn apart because of money worries and the best way to safeguard yourself from this is to instil a culture of financial modesty in the home. It is all very well and good to keep a nice comfortable home, but if your finances are spread too thin and the new 55-inch TV dominates a cold room because the heating bill is unpaid, then things are going awry.

The household kitty is a monthly budget that should be very transparent between the husband and wife, and respected by the children. There are many good books out there on how best to deal with personal finance and the financial running of the home, which can and should be further researched, but for the sake of common sense your most important expenses should be considered and consistent and include the following:

Critical financial obligations in order of priority:

- Ensure the mortgage or rent is paid on time.
- Heating and electricity bills take priority over mobile phone and entertainment expenses such as supplemented TV channels.
- Ensure there is enough food in the house to keep your family sustained and healthy. It needn't be expensive or fancy, but it needs to be enough.
- Ensure that insurances are in place and valid. To include life insurance, household and if applicable, motor insurance. Being without this trinity of insurances leaves you vulnerable against the cruelties of life which are beyond your control.
- Savings. How much is up to you but a good idea is to build up an emergency fund before saving for the 'fun stuff'. An emergency fund to comfortably sustain all (critical) family expenses for at least three months is a smart way to buffer your family against job loss or illness. Nothing is certain in life and protection against what the tides may bring is common sense*. Keep it in an easy to access savings account or in premium bonds.
- Expenses for commuting to work or school.
- Debt payments. Make the minimum payment in times of lack, but do make them.

*If you have emergency savings in place for unforeseen circumstances it will bring about a sense of wellbeing and a feeling of security within your marriage and household. Feeling in control of your finances regardless of what the future may bring is empowering. Financial angst is the top cause of stress for over 40% of adults. Don't conform to the pattern of this world. Financial freedom makes you far richer in spirit than what any tangible 'object' can give you.

All other expenses are not of critical priority and should be the first to go if you find yourself in financial difficulty, these include:

- Gym memberships.
- TV and movie subscriptions.
- Extra curricular activities and paid club memberships.
- Entertainment and eating out.

- Non-essential clothing items. Only buy if an item requires replacing and is critical such as warm jackets for winter, or outgrown/worn out shoes for the children.
- Beauty treatments, including haircuts.
- Birthday and Christmas gifts for extended family and friends, they'll understand.
- Replacement of household goods.

If things are getting on top of you seek help from a charity such as CAP UK or a national, government-backed (most importantly, free) debt advice service.

Have casual and dependable rituals in the home

Nothing says home and belonging more than a few family rituals. This could be anything from a special Saturday breakfast to 'board game night' on a Friday. Perhaps you could make Sunday a 'family only' day and enjoy a whopping great feast and it is absolutely imperative that all immediate family members attend.

Rituals could include:

- A luxurious bubble bath on a given night of the week per family member —no trespassing!
- Favourite dinner night. One night of the week a family member gets to choose his/her favourite dinner. Turns are taken per family member, per week.
- Gourmet night. Choose a special dish to make that you have never tried before and get the family involved in the cooking and preparation.
- A story in the 'big bed' before bedtime for the younger children on a suitable day. All family members attend in their pyjamas and take turns to read a page.
- Board Game or puzzle night. Parents get a night off cooking and order a takeaway. No television allowed.
- Setting the table for Sunday lunch with the children and letting them choose who sits where.
- Post-Sunday breakfast walk in the country, or your nearest outdoor green space.
- Movie matinee Saturday (at the cinema or at home). Popcorn and chocolates included.

- Leave prettily wrapped chocolates or cookies on a neighbours doorstep. Knock on their door and run as fast as you can home! Everyone is under strict instructions to never give the game away and expose your family as the secret gifters.

The familiarity of home breeds a sense of belonging and stability, and when the atmosphere is stable, so is the mood and the manners. Especially when it comes to the children.

Make and enjoy family traditions

The traditions of your home and family will largely depend on your personal interests and culture, and that is exactly what makes life richer. Having familiar traditions and the 'way you do things' are what makes home feel like home and provides a sense of belonging for all. My family are of Danish heritage and where possible we honour that. Dancing around the Christmas tree singing loud songs is very alien to outsiders and newcomers to the fold, but to us it is one of the highlights of the season. Memories of seeing my somewhat stoic and shy family stumbling around a tree and fumbling for the words to festive songs makes me smile and fills me with a deep love and appreciation for them.

If you find yourself struggling to think of your own personal traditions, then make some! How you run your household with your spouse is yours for the creating, and that's what makes having a family and homemaking ever so special.

This extra attention and thoughtfulness into making your house a home are what bind a family together. Where there is love, belonging, togetherness and a little shared time, there makes a happy household held in high regard by all.

Enjoy your home and make it comfortable

We are not given a rule book for our home life and the operation of our houses. Many fall prey to the consumer trap, told how our homes should be decorated and what we should possess within our four walls. In the long run this only breeds discontent and takes your focus away from creating a *heart* for your home. Never allow your culture to dictate what feels comfortable to you in your home. The home and your enjoyment of it should be of paramount importance to you and your family. Fret not if your kitchen is old and out of 'style'. So long as it is kept orderly and hygienic, and is a place where you lovingly prepare meals to nourish your family is what matters. The same goes for the style of your sofa, the size of your TV and the colour of your walls. Do what makes *you* feel happy and try to ignore the world and what it's selling. After all, it is only you and your family who reside within your address so make it wonderful for you, however you define that.

There are billions of households on this earth and not all of them are going to look like the cover of an interiors magazine. Worry less about using it as a status symbol and concentrate on the people inside it more.

Home is not a word for 'a brick built box of things', it is a place of feeling and contentment, pleasure, belonging, togetherness, and love. No matter how aesthetically pleasing the interior may be, if the house is not filled with laughter and love it is merely a pretty shell.

Instilling the English values of what home *truly* means will release you from the trappings of modern expectations and give your home a timeless feel that people will want to return to again and again. It's less about the furnishings and more about the connection, relationship and behaviour of the people who reside behind that front door.

Put etiquette into practice

There is no greater time than the present to put what you are learning into practice, and none more so than in times of domestic stress and dispute. Your household may be used to bickering, poor manners, or living in a state of 'mess', but if you wish to make a difference to the feel of your home and change the attitudes of the people within it you must practice daily. Habits do not form instantly, so choose to take a positive step in transforming your family and home into a beacon of light and happiness.

Etiquette means to put yourself and others at ease. No individual under your roof will be able to demonstrate their understanding of this in the outside world, *unless* they are doing so at home. To recap the very basics of homegrown etiquette:

- Your management of the home reflects the state of your mind, keep it in order.
- Uphold and respect the authority for the head of the household.
- Remember that parents make the rules and children must abide by them.
- The art of discipline and the development of good character begins at home.
- Everyone should help to maintain the household (according to age, no one is exempt).

- Respect the things in your home. No slamming doors, or abusing inanimate objects.
- Have respect for other people's belongings and personal space.
- Show respect to your neighbours.
- You **are** your family, work together, uphold the family name.
- Above all, love one another, with all your might.

SOCIAL SUCCESS & SOIRÉES

SOCIAL & REPUTATION MANAGEMENT

Measured by what we say, and what we do

Graces are skills that we use to interact politely in all social situations, whether at home with your family or spouse, at a party with friends, or in a public place with a thousand strangers. We all need social graces in order to get along.

Many people lack knowledge of social graces and etiquette and while some 'lessons' are exclusive to men and some to women, there are a variety of rules that we all must adhere to if we are to get along. Some think many of these rules and standards are archaic and no longer apply, but these are often the same people who don't like to comply to *any* rules and would gladly see society degrade into a culture of self-serving individuals who are only interested in how they can get ahead rather than how they can get along.

All women who wish to become ladies should learn, appreciate and apply social graces wherever they may go. It's what sets a lady apart and she knows this. All men who wish to be gentlemen will set aside his testosterone fuelled behaviour and desire for oneupmanship in order to make his comrades feel at ease and his lady always well protected.

Social graces are universally appreciated and should be exercised at all times.

Take care however to ensure that your motivation for learning these skills is for the right reasons.

You can meet plenty of beguilers who put on plummy accents, but the glossy exterior which blinds you with deception will be unravelled the moment they are rude to a waiter, or decide to verbally put you down for something you said or did. No true English lady or gent would entertain such a pretender. We are obliged to remain true, faithful and genuine. That goes for our personal conviction and those we wish to surround ourselves with. Attitude rubs off, and we want ours protected.

What might appear to be aloofness at first from the English is just a form of sniffing you out. Do you genuinely appreciate our company and personality, or are you social climbing? In order to truly fit in you must leave behind not only the opinion of 'hoi pilloi' (the masses), but lay aside any aspiration of making yourself financially rich or famous through association.

This rule does not only apply to the royal, aristocratic, upper or middle classes, but to all levels of social standing and financial solvency within the British class system. If you are, indeed truly English in your way of life this moral compass strongly applies. We have no time for fools and pretenders. Your manners may take you places, but your heart and your reputation are what keep you there. Our reputation in association with yours is what we truly care about, as well as having a cracking life-long, trust-filled friendship.

We hate to be embarrassed, and *especially* by association.

Always remember that there is little else the English are particularly fond of than protecting their reputation and their dignity. This is probably why so many satires and television shows have us putting on these 'airs and graces', it keeps less desirable people at a safe distance. There is truth in it of course, but certainly no malice.

In an archaic sense, the English will critique you in order to establish whether you are a threat to the tribe. It goes without saying that first impressions upon meeting count, and so does reputation. Even if you might make a less than favourable impression in the beginning, you can with improved dignity and hard effort usually win someone round, but continued unsavoury behaviour counts as a permanent black mark. We are a very polite bunch but there is only so much we can take. I'm the first to admit that it is terribly taxing to be nice to people all the time, especially when you are having a bad day, or perhaps find a person and their behaviour distasteful, but why let that sully you?

Therefore how you come across matters *all the time*, not just upon the first meeting.

Some may argue that they don't care about people's opinions and their reputations. Don't believe them, or adopt their viewpoint. We are *built* to care what people think about us, else, why is this book written, and why are you reading it?

Here, we'll look at the core elements of what makes for a 'good reputation', analyse the common pitfalls people encounter, and what you can do to manage, maintain and spruce up your character at any stage.

Manners Come as Standard

Greeting and first meeting

Now considered an old fashioned way of greeting a new acquaintance, saying, "How do you do, I am (insert name here)" might seem something only the Queen would say, but it is still the *correct* way of greeting someone you have never met before. Formalities still have their place and are at times, really useful. For instance, how do you *know* it is nice, or if you are 'pleased' to meet someone? They could turn out to be a horror within two minutes. Save yourself the embarrassment of a gushing first greeting and err on the side of caution. Once the initial greeting is out of the way, you may follow up later with "I have heard so much about you and have been looking forward to meeting you", to soften the formality if you wish.

It is acceptable to offer a much warmer greeting if you have exchanged contact via email or telephone with your acquaintance before meeting face to face.

Note that the question of "How do you do?" is always a rhetorical one, you do not answer it with anything but an identical response, including the introduction of your name. A new acquaintance need not hear about your motor troubles/digestive issues/bad mood. If you feel "How do you do?" is still too formal for your taste, replace this greeting with a simple "Hello".

A kinder upper hand

Upon greeting a new acquaintance, it is customary to do so with a handshake. The English are not all that keen on continental 'air-kissing' with new blood, though it is becoming commonplace as time marches on and European forms of etiquette are brought into the fold. English gentlemen are still required to offer a hand, to both fellow men and ladies alike, but if his female company is well known he may oblige with a kiss on the cheek if she offers hers.

Ladies greeting strangers should offer a hand, not a cheek. This rule can be relaxed when you know your company on a more intimate level. One should never offer a cheek kiss upon the first meeting, no matter how much you have heard about the person from a good friend. If the new acquaint offers first, then oblige so as not to make them feel uncomfortable. Thrusting your hand out for a shake instead of leaning in the for the kiss is a slap in the face of someone wishing to break the ice with you.

With regard to continental cheek kisses, let it be said that you never actually make contact with the other person's face with your lips, instead, merely a brush of the fleshy part of your cheek against the other persons will suffice. Noisy 'lip smack' sounds are also unnecessary. Steel yourself also for the 'double cheek kiss'. It's always hard to tell if someone is a one or two cheek kisser, so posture yourself and play it by ear. Neither hover for that second kiss, or pull away too fast. As hard as it may be to be so close to a strange body, try and relax into the encounter.

It is of the utmost importance, cheek kissing or not, that your hands must be in their right place at all times. It is politer to gently grasp the upper arms of your greeting partner, or at elbow level when going in for a kiss. Strictly **no** touching of the bust or chest, the waist or anywhere below including the bottom, the small of the back, the very tops of the shoulders, or too near the face. Note that this kiss must also never be too near to the corner of the mouth, or lips be involved at all. It is merely a meeting of cheek-to-cheek that is considered acceptable.

The custom of shaking hands has its roots in medieval times. The world was as unsavoury and dangerous in those times as it is now, and people often concealed weapons (have times really changed? Though now it's more attitude and a sharp tongue, than pistols). The expression of a handshake would demonstrate you were not hiding a weapon, or wish to cause harm. It also demonstrates your trust in the other person, and puts you on equal footing. To refuse to shake someone's hand is as offensive today as it would have been hundreds of years ago. Though a dagger may not be present at the time of modern insult, the wound left over is just as deep. Regardless of your preconceived ideas about someone, always shake their hand. With that in mind, always offer to shake the hand of a known foe too, it disarms them in more than just a physical sense.

Note that handshakes must be firm but not bone-crushing. Limp 'wet fish' handshakes are an instant turn off and will not be forgotten in a hurry. Ladies should shake hands like men, the *quality* of a handshake is gender neutral. If a lady offers her hand as if expecting you to kiss it this will be deemed social suicide on her part. Utterly distasteful to be *that* woman. No one is 'above' the practice of a common handshake. Two and no more than three lively and pleasingly firm 'pumps' are all that is required for a handshake and under **no** circumstances should you include your left hand into the mix. Males in particular like to demonstrate their social status by clasping over another man's hand or 'supporting' the handshake by holding the underside of his fellow's arm. This is an embarrassingly obvious way of showing you are desperate to be top-dog and is a social turn off. Regardless of whether you are socially superior (in your not-so humble opinion), you are *always* meeting an equal.

Remember to shake hands upon leaving as well as arrival. Social air kissing with new acquaintances is considered *slightly* more acceptable upon leaving than greeting, but still tread carefully with that one.

Eye contact

It goes without saying that whenever you greet or are introduced to someone, you must look that person in the eye and maintain good eye contact through the entire engagement. Work on cultivating a pleasant level of eye contact as eye-balling a person without breaking your gaze from time to time can be off-putting too. Especially if you are standing too close.

Personal space

When involved in a standing introduction, you may lean in ever so slightly to shake a hand but make sure you are never closer to that person than a slightly-bent arm's length. Sixty centimeters is ideal. Stood too near it becomes suffocating and restricts the ability for your partner to circulate when he tires of you, stood too far back and you appear disengaged.

A valued name

A person's name means so much more to the individual than a sequence of letters on paper that identifies them. A name is very much a *part* of our identity, and as such you must make it a priority to learn, remember and know how to pronounce names correctly. If, like the author you were in receipt of a hard to pronounce moniker at birth, or by marriage, you must have enough self-respect to demand people call you by the correct name and not some wishy-washy offshoot. Correction may seem awkward but you'll be glad you requested it in the end. I have lost count of the amount of times people have called me Elaine. I do not remember those people fondly.

It is most disrespectful to not make an effort on the pronunciation of a name. A substitute will never 'do'. If you have to ask several times, then do it. Better the initial annoyance and hard work then forever losing respect because you simply couldn't be bothered to learn, or were too shy to ask again. Worse yet to continually get it wrong.

It is also good manners to address and introduce older generations by their title and surname rather than their christian names, it is a subtle way to show respect and gives them the option to ask you to address them by first name. It is of their choosing whether or not they offer up their first name to a new acquaintance.

When introducing yourself to anyone for the first time, ideally do so by your first and last name. If you lead with your first name, follow with the surname.

If you find yourself in an uneasy social situation or wish to keep a little anonymity in public it is also perfectly acceptable to introduce yourself and ask to be addressed by title and surname only. Your christian name is one of the final steps in giving over almost your whole identity in this modern age so it is fine to guard it with your life if you feel it necessary among unfamiliar company.

Remembering names is sometimes difficult. Try to link some part of their personality or appearance to a mental picture of the person and the said name. For example "Julie likes pearl jewellery", or "Martin drives a Mercedes". You may have to dig a little to find a tidbit of information you can latch to the name. But for goodness sake keep these little lyrics in your head, and do not mutter them aloud.

If all else fails, then confess you have forgotten a person's name. My oft used phrase is, "I'm very sorry, I am great with faces but terrible with names, what is it again?" When they tell you, say "That's it. So sorry. How was your trip to Italy/how are your children?". Then make sure to remember their name this time! Follow up this trifle with positive conversation and the matter will be closed.

Reputations rest upon names, make sure to get it right!

Please and thank you

It goes without saying that remembering to use your pleases and thank yous all the time is the holy grail of good manners and reputation. No proper lady or gentleman would even consider omitting these basics when interacting with a fellow person, regardless of their 'perceived importance' or lack thereof. It is a telltale sign of one who is 'playing up' to their company and wearing airs and graces when they are kind to the host but not the help.

In a restaurant or any type of service setting, you should care as much about making your waiter/service provider feel as valued as the company you are with.

Your children also demonstrate how high a value the parent places on common courtesies, and though young children are often forgetful, to not say please and thank you in front of the parent and it *not* be corrected immediately says more about the parent than it does the child. Remind your children and drum in the importance of saying please and thank you at every opportunity.

Entering a room or an event

You may have been told your entire early adult life by the media and certain social 'experts' that in order to appear socially confident you must make a show stopping entrance to any party. Be noticed, they say. The more glitter, trumpets and ostrich feathers the better, but to the English this idea is nothing short of horrifying.

Gone are the days of being announced into a society party or royal court, and so instead you must marry the art of slipping into a soirée without too much fuss yet balancing this quiet arrival without becoming a complete wallflower.

Upon arrival at any event, should they not be there to greet you in the first instance, your first priority is to find your host. This is to announce your arrival, thank them immediately for the invitation, pass on any gift or offering you may have taken with you and allow your host to do with you as they please. More often than not your host may have someone in mind they wish to introduce you to, this also happily negates the need for you to painfully introduce yourself to anyone who appears to be unoccupied.

Whatever you do, never stand around like a lemon. Make yourself busy by either finding your host, putting away your outerwear, delivering a bottle of wine to the bar, or heading there to grab a refreshment. Push yourself to enter the throng of the crowd and you will soon find yourself in the swing of things. Standing against a wall as if thrust there by centrifugal force will only make you look uneasy and a social bore.

The art of small talk

Small talk is a fine art, an accomplishment at which some excel, namely ladies, while others offer only dry and awkward drivel. The key to get the conversation in motion is to think ahead of an event what you might ask, or how you may be linked to someone socially. For example;

"I hear that you and Michael play tennis together. How long have you been playing?"

Or, for those less familiar on your radar;

"How do you know the Middletons?"

Whenever you make small talk it must heavily feature light, open-ended and easy to answer questions so that the conversation flows and your company has something with which to respond at length.

Comments about the weather, flat opinions and what seems like a friendly "Lovely evening isn't it?", usually follow with nothing but a response of a sigh, wry smile, a nod, or one word reply.

The absolute key with successful small talk and making a good impression is to allow your company to talk about themselves as much as possible. People love nothing more than to talk about themselves and doing so provides you with more tidbits with which to lead and develop the conversation further.

A good tip for making friends easily is to answer any questions about yourself with an enquiry for the opinion of your chatting partner, or any common ground you may have. For instance, you may be talking about your latest skiing holiday, so impart a few light facts about where you stayed or what you did, then ask your new friend if they like to ski, or if not, "Have they ever considered it, for it is a wonderful way to spend an early spring getaway. Where do you like to holiday?" You have offered a hobby of yours, given them a tip on where to stay and shown interest in what *they* like to do in a very short monologue. Off they go again talking about themselves and providing you with more facts to work with.

Sleuthing for lighthearted facts about someone and what they like to do makes it a breeze introducing this new friend to someone you might already know. "Maria, this is Janet, she enjoys wine tasting too. Where did you say you holidayed last Janet, was it Umbria?" I think you get the picture?

If you wish to depart from the company of a guest who is boring you to tears you have three vaguely polite options:

1. Excuse yourself to use the bathroom, saying "Would you please excuse me, I just need to pop to the ladies/gents". Then go and use it, or at least

appear to. Being overly concerned as to what you or others call the lavatory/loo/toilet/bog/little girl's/boy's room is pure snobbery and no longer realistic. Simply "Ladies" or "Gents" will do, a neutral turn of phrase that is clearly understood and still savoury in its description.

2. A better option is to offer to collect a top-up or drink. Likely they will refuse your offer, but if they accept then go and collect a drink for them but 'bump into' someone on the way. Tell the person you collected a drink for that it has been lovely chatting but you must catch up with "XYZ". Hand them their drink and make a swift exit. Should your glass be full when you wish to make your escape then cough awkwardly a few times and announce you are going "I'm sorry I must go in search of a glass of water, can I get you anything whilst I'm there?". Make sure not to return too soon.

3. Introduce them to someone else, give a little fuel to spark their conversation then make your excuses to visit the gents/get a glass of water/step out for air. Not entirely fair on the person you introduced but this is the game Brits play best. It's called 'pass the bore'. You all must play your part in the game and take one for the team, for at least a little time during the party. The aim is to not get stuck for too long but make sure that the boring guest feels appreciated all the same.

See: Making Polite Conversation for small talk subjects that can lead to social suicide.

Mingling

See point above regarding small talk, after a polite amount of time making chit-chat kindly make your excuse to move on. Find new 'victim'. Rinse and repeat.

Leaving a room or party

Never leave a party without thanking your hosts and bidding them farewell. To disappear without trace from a party is bad form. If you must make a sly and hopefully unnoticed exit (usually due to an overestimated ability to imbibe), send a short text message to your friend or ask a close friend also at the party to make apologies for you. Then you must follow up the next day with some form of communication to apologise for your ungraceful exit.

It is personal choice as to whether you say goodbye to everyone at a large party, but bear in mind you will likely be interrupting conversations. Do not expect those with whom you are saying farewell to stop their conversation entirely. Politely touch them on the shoulder or forearm and say, "Sorry for interrupting, I just wanted to say a quick goodbye, we must catch up, farewell". If you know them well and meant this gesture then follow up within two days. If they are a new acquaintance and you would like to remain in touch, hand them a social card.

See: Social Graces - Correspondence and Stationery, for details on social cards.

At a smaller gathering such as a dinner party, it would be impolite to leave without saying goodbye to all. If all guests are within one room you can do this at once by announcing to the room that you had a great time, hope they have a wonderful evening and wish them all well. Then make your exit, do not hang on for longer than necessary.

MAKING POLITE CONVERSATION

Conversation is a wide and varied subject, as to be expected. Therefore it is hard to narrow down any rules and regulations on what makes good conversation, but we can at the very least discuss what is *impolite*. Your manner of discussion says a lot about your morals, values and personal boundaries, so therefore try to always keep things light and positive when talking in the company of people you don't know. You would be hard-pushed to make any real friends without talking about some nitty gritty things, so go ahead and forge lasting friendships when the timing is right, but when in new or strange company and especially on formal occasions, beware of the following subjects:

Money

It is never polite to discuss money in any form while in a social setting. Any financial issues that need to be resolved between friends, business associates, or family should be done so privately. One should certainly never ask a friend how much they earn, how much they spent on something, or get into a discussion surrounding the wealth of other people. It is also vulgar to boast about how much you earn, the value of your possessions, or the profit made on a deal.

Be aware also of your own tongue and what it declares subtly, try not to imply that you do or *do not* have money. Never complain about being 'poor' as you may view it. There are always people in a worse situation than you are and they will be making personal judgments about what you drive, are wearing, or where you live that could make them feel terrible about themselves. Your finances are of no-ones concern and can make people feel rather uncomfortable. The only people to discuss them with are your spouse, business partner, accountant, and bank manager. Try also to not declare even in a joking way, that you are "broke", or wouldn't be able to afford something that someone else has. You never know, fortunes change, and be mindful that when you declare such things people will always make an assumption about your financial situation and those opinions stick. Keep the topic of your bank balance *private*.

Should someone ask you for financial advice, gladly help if you are able, or it's a subject in which you are particularly knowledgeable or have experience in.

Insist that it is conducted at a dedicated time rather than at a dinner party, over a casual drink, or coffee, and certainly never done 'on the spot'. The subject of someones finances and the advice you impart should be treated with respect, kept strictly professional, and above all, private.

Divorce

Divorce is a sad fact of life—to some devastating, and to others, liberating. Avoid discussions regarding divorces unless you are acting in support of a friend, but be mindful of not allowing yourself to get wrapped up in the drama of the situation. Instead try to remain neutral, impartial and advise only on practical matters. Speak about it in private too, you never know who may be listening in.

You are there to be a listening and comforting ear, not an opinionated gossip partner.

When a couple are divorcing, passions often rise and spiteful things are said. Try to take everything with a pinch of salt and distance yourself from the situation if at all possible. Incredibly hurtful things are sometimes said and done and the last thing you want is to get yourself or your immediate family wrapped up in the drama. By all means, support a friend who is having a tough time emotionally but remain pragmatic and refuse to say nasty things about the other party.

Separated couples sometimes reconcile. Your unkind words or opinions won't easily be forgotten by either party. You may also have differing moral opinions on divorce, do not judge the couple but instead speak only words of hope and positivity. You needn't sprinkle any opinions, judgment or negativity on this already sad situation.

Disputes with neighbours

Not everyone is blessed with good and gracious neighbours. Many people find themselves in a terrible battle regarding noise, property, and general clashes of lifestyle that only serve to tear apart communities. If you have a dispute that you feel is having a detrimental affect on your wellbeing and standards of living then by all means approach your local authority for advice but in every circumstance do not discuss neighbourly disputes with fellow neighbours or friends unless you are actively asking them to bear witness for the cause of legal involvement.

Gossip, threats and spiteful talk will only give rise to a dispute and ultimately means you lose control of a situation. Whenever there is conflict with a neighbour never lower yourself to a shouting match or acting spitefully. Neighbourly disputes can cause violence and send people in a tailspin. The one place you are meant to feel safe is at home so do not give malicious thoughts or deeds the time of day. You stand in better stead with the authorities if you remain calm and note down the date and time of any incidences and act upon them pragmatically. Your wellbeing and mental health will be better placed if you stay in control. No one wants to be the 'bad neighbour', take the higher ground in all situations.

Disputes with friends

They are inevitable, unless you allows insult to just slide right off, you are bound to have a falling out or a dispute with a friend sometime in this journey of life. With such variety in morals, politics, opinions, and lifestyle choices not everyone will fit your mould and it is easy to feel rubbed up the wrong way sometimes. The marker of a lady or a gentleman is how he or she handles offence, what he or she does *not* do in response, and most certainly what he or she says about it to others.

There are people who are passionate, fiery and downright self-righteous. These are the types who will aggressively tell you what's on their mind (whether they are right or wrong), and there are those who never say anything directly to you but like to tell all and sundry (especially the internet) about how awful you are. There are two ways in which you can handle these situations but only one will do *your* reputation any good.

Firstly, you can approach the situation head on and have it out with your opponent **in private**. Be warned, that the moment you raise your voice, accuse, blame or deny any involvement in the 'issue' then you have lost any chance of resolving the situation. True maturity is humbling yourself but doing so with integrity. Admit your wrongdoing, or whatever you may have done that has caused offence and apologise for either the action, or simply the stalemate you both find yourselves in.

Do not shout. Accusing, berating, shaming and harassing rarely gets you anywhere and is no way to salvage a friendship, so you must take the higher ground. In order to keep your dignity intact you must remain calm, refuse to moan or gossip about ex-friends and remain steadfast in your humility. If it cannot be sorted quietly between the two of you, then there is little hope and it is of no use getting a third party involved.

The alternative is to move on. Be careful with your desire to set the record straight, seek revenge or show the rest of the world how nasty someone is. Revenge and spite only ever reflects poorly on the person dishing it up and is great reason for your foe to seek sympathy from others, and turning *you* into the bad guy.

No Englishman or woman would be caught dead giving a foe the time of day, or be caught gossiping about them. Paint on that stiff upper lip and move on.

Most importantly, ask yourself what you can learn from the experience. Do you tend to fall out with people after a while? Use these negative experiences as a way to gain insight as to who you are willing to spend your time with and what kind of person you attract into your life. Are there patterns that need altering? Friends that do not bring positive experiences and feelings into your life? Are there some destructive or desperate behaviours going on in your life? You may find some common themes and similarities in the type of person you entertain and how soon you embrace them without knowing who they really are.

Try and raise the bar in your standard of friends, staying away from gossips and those seeking to be spiteful, it's the best way to protect yourself in the future.

Never, gossip about your friends, or someone else's. It's a simple rule, but one hard to live by—try your hardest and do it anyway!

Never, ever fight in public. Silence is golden, even when someone is mocking, shouting or outright insulting you in the street. Not that I wish for you to ever be in that situation, but if you ever are, grit your teeth, walk away and pat yourself on the back for having an ounce of grace and classier civic manners.

Lawsuits

Like money, divorce, and cat-fights, to discuss lawsuits in public with someone other than your legal representative is poor taste. You never know who may be listening in on the conversation, especially when the issues you are discussing are highly sensitive and confidential. Make it one of your personal scruples and refuse to discuss lawsuits in which you are not directly involved or can offer sound legal advice. Conversations regarding law should also be conducted in a professional setting.

Politics

Unless you find yourself in a relevant setting, politics should not be discussed in any great detail or length at a social occasion. There is a time for politics and the last place it should be considered a conversation topic are at celebrations, in a business setting, or in any establishment or private home where alcohol is being consumed. To converse about politics with anything other than a sober mind is to invite disaster. Never ask a person directly who they voted for, or will vote for in an upcoming election. That is as much your business as their inside leg measurement. There is a reason voting is done so privately, respect that. Should you ever find yourself in an uncomfortable situation where debate is rather heated, do not be afraid to speak up and ask that the subject be changed. If the parties refuse to stop, then calmly leave the room or remove yourself from the conversation entirely. In these situations, to remove yourself from instances whereby you feel uncomfortable is completely acceptable. Never rise to a jibe or come to the defence about a party or candidate you vote for. A poker face is your strongest asset. Leave the fighting to the politicians. Their time in the sun rarely lasts beyond a season anyway, choose not to lose friends over it.

Health

Medical and illness related conversation (particularly in a negative light) is never a pretty subject to discuss in public. Think of your surroundings, particularly in eating establishments. Strangers *do not* want to hear about the maladies of your body or anyone else's for that matter. Discuss health-giving therapies and tinctures by all means, but complain not about ailments or discuss gruesome details.

Religion, not to be confused with faith

Spirituality, faith, and hope make nice conversation when discussed with love and respect, but be aware the trap of falling into dialogue about religious condemnation and 'rules'. If people should ask you details about your spiritual persuasion this is a subject best discussed, or debated, in private.

This is a difficult subject to approach even in writing as a person's beliefs are individual, but let it be known, no person of true faith will ever share their beliefs with you with the aim of stifling your life or sapping the joy from it. They are simply trying to share a passion and a purpose that has enriched their life, so do not come against it in anger. To do so is to invalidate their feelings in order to appear 'right', a personality trait which is never appealing.

Feel free to disagree, but respectfully so. Should a conversation about faith or belief make you feel uncomfortable, then let your companions know quietly and politely. The other person will and should respect your wishes. In a group setting where they are discussing faith, simply walk away or remove yourself from the conversation if you feel uneasy. Free speech is a right available to all, if you don't want to hear it then move away. To tear apart someone's opinion, and wish to publicly humiliate another person because of their faith or beliefs is self-righteous and unattractive.

'Religion' with its legalistic, overbearing rules might come against you, but people with surrendered *faith* will not. Any believer of a scriptural faith will instinctively know that they should respect your wishes and not rise to anger or pride. They are known by their 'fruit' and that is seen in their compassion, respect for others, understanding and acceptance that we are all different.

LESSONS IN INTEGRITY

Do what you say you'll do

Half the battle of earning and keeping respect from those around you is centred around your character, integrity, and honesty. One of the surest ways to keep standards high is to simply do as you say you'll do. If you make a promise, keep it. This goes for the promise to your spouse to remain faithful. The promise to your employer to turn up to work and do what he is paying you to do. The promise to your landlord or mortgage provider to make your payments on time. The promise to your children to love, care and protect them, and to stand by the tiniest of daily promises you make every day.

Care about your character, and keep your integrity in good order.

Celebrate other people's blessings

Be careful who you share good news with. It is unfortunate that not everyone will be happy for you. There are some personalities who do not wish to see or hear of positive things which do not directly involve or benefit them. Negative people who might surround you will often try to bring down your successes. This is not under your control of course, but if you refrain from sharing information with these people then you cannot become a victim of their tear-down schemes. Be modest, careful and considered with whom you share personal information and good news.

Search your heart and question whether you are one of these people yourself. If you find you cannot be happy for even your closest friends when things go right for them then you must evaluate your ability to conduct supportive relationships. Negative living is a choice we make, and if you believe in the idiom that 'you get what you give', then who would want to send out negative and jealous vibes into the atmosphere? Though it can be hard, you must swallow your jealousy and desire to compare your life with others. Your reputation and relationships will suffer in the long run if your friends and family do not want to share their good news and blessings with you. Being supportive, positive and the ability to be happy for other people is a blessing in its own right.

You must do what you can to help other people reach their goals as you never know when you might need the favour returned. Make recommendations, be helpful and kind to those who seek your advice, most of all be encouraging. Though you might not be able to help someone directly with their goals, you can help them indirectly through words of encouragement, praise, and by uplifting them whenever you meet.

Share the limelight and share praise

Living in a culture that promotes a 'me first' attitude, we are not automatically programmed to praise others. Instead we are encouraged to want to come first, be the best, be the winner, the top dog. Acting like this at work may get you far but won't win you many friends.

In order to win friends, and more importantly keep them, it is a safer bet to share the limelight and praise with those deserving of it. Recognise, acknowledge and share with those around you the talents, strengths and achievements of your peers.

This is especially crucial at work. In order to be esteemed as a team player, you must take on tasks and share rewards as a team.

Look the part

There is a whole module later in this book on the nuances of dressing politely and well enough to give a good impression. Your wardrobe choices, reputation and self-esteem are interlinked. Further details can be found at length in the chapters on personal appearance. Just take note that it matters to your reputation to follow the guidance laid out. Three basic rules to remember are:

- Be clean
- Be modest
- Be nondescript

Be strict with your online presence

There is a very real concern over the correlation of our use of social media and our levels of self-esteem. To be frank, social media isn't much use to anyone unless they are selling a product, stalking someone, or wish to get caught in the trap of seeking validation from strangers. Agreed, it can be lovely to connect with people and see all those 'likes and comments', and there are some lovely sides to social media, but countless psychological studies have shown that spending large amounts of time on these platforms can have a serious negative impact on your mental health. So if you must use it, be conscious of the time you spend and the negative impact it could be having on your mental wellbeing and *real* social life as a result. Is it stealing time from you and your family? Are you updating your status or adding pictures online to impress complete strangers? Do those likes give you a little 'boost'? If so, evaluate, and *feel free to delete your accounts*. There is no law, (aside from the social pressures of current culture), that says you must have a presence on social media.

If it makes you feel uncomfortable in any way or you don't know why you are on there, then delete those online accounts. Your family will still know you, and your friends will still hang out with you. Promise. You might surprise yourself by having something new and interesting to talk about when you next see each other as you won't have had the 'social media heads-up'. Now there's a thought!

Social media can be damaging to relationships and friendships given the amount of time a person invests staring into their screens as opposed to spending real, valuable time with loved ones and in the physical presence of others. Considering how 'connected' we are in this day and age, life has never felt more lonely. Step away from the 'me' culture that surrounds social media and take the higher ground. If the Queen doesn't have a Facebook account, tweet insults (here's looking at you Trump), or Instagram her breakfast then why did *we* ever think it was cool?

Employers are now wise enough to search your name on the internet to see what they find before they interview you or offer you a position, potential romantic partners can do this too. If you wouldn't be happy for it to appear on the six o'clock news, then why post it on the internet? Wouldn't it be lovely to have a little 'air of mystery' surrounding your daily comings and goings?

Your world won't end by shutting those accounts down, but it'll be a whole lot richer and in the moment! Nothing is classier, or shows more strength of character than a person who refuses to conform to trends—social media being one of them.

PUBLIC CONDUCT

You are what you drink

We all like a tipple now and again. The English are especially known for their ability to put away the booze, but what separates the best of the crop from common boozers is an individual's self-control and knowing the right place and time to imbibe. It cannot be denied that we have a *very* strong drinking culture in England, which is sadly known to be more than a little undignified.

To 'enjoy' a drink is to appreciate the drink itself, not the drunkenness. The heritage, story and artisan method in which wines, beers, ales and spirits were created should be something more of us appreciate. To indulge in a little personal education regarding your favourite drink will help you in the long run, not only in the booze aisle, but in your attitude and how you relate to and respect alcohol. There are many fine English producers and equally fine importers of quality alcohol that are wonderful to savour, appreciate and enjoy but if one would like to be known as an upstanding English lady or gentleman they must *refrain* from drinking cheap booze for the sake of it. It is, after all, considered incredibly 'common'.

Pubs are the foundation of our British social scene. Unsurprisingly there are a *variety* of ales, ciders and beers to enjoy as well as imported wines selected by the landlord or sommelier. These beverages aren't just there to get you in an unfit state to walk, they are there to be revered.

When you accept an invitation to a pub or bar, if you choose to drink alcohol (yes, you have a *choice*), make sure to spend time studying the variety on offer, order according to taste and enjoy the drink as opposed to 'downing it'. If you treat alcohol with respect, it will in turn respect you. One expensive and highly enjoyable glass of wine is worth far more to the experience than ordering the cheapest bottle to 'drain' for the sake of acting inappropriately, getting more for your money, and feeling spectacularly rough the following day.

Drinking what you consider to be a 'luxury', slowly, and with great care allows you to stay in control and view the occasion as a treat. Better that than looking like you are desperately trying to hydrate yourself after a trip to the desert. This is England after all, rarely are we *that* hot or parched after the marathon tea drinking that goes on all day. So for goodness sake, slow down!

In English culture, drinking socially with friends is considered a weekend pastime. We may go to the pub on a Friday or Saturday evening, but we mostly socialise in each other's homes and gardens. Drinking at home is more economical financially, but one must still bring their fair share to the party. Behaviour is often better managed in a safe environment such as the home but this is no reason to let your guard down. Passing out, or worse, vomiting from too much drink is as unattractive behind closed doors as it is in the street.

Social studies have proven that a group's behaviour when drunk is based entirely upon the cultural *assumption* of what alcohol does to you. Essentially, this means that it is all in the mind. If you expect yourself to become aggressive, crude, flirtatious, angry and prone to violence, then you will be. If you expect to 'chill out', be more cheerful and peaceful then this is more likely the outcome you will experience. You can even 'think yourself' tipsy. The brain works like a computer, if you put yourself in a social setting where a certain type of behaviour is expected then the memory bank in your brain will bring forth the expected behaviour associated with drinking alcohol.

This makes sense when you think of the times you have consumed alcohol but haven't felt entirely in the mood and as if the alcohol has had no effect. This is also true of solo drinking, you may feel the *physical* effects of the alcohol, but it's a bit less 'fun' than when drinking with friends.

Regardless of your opinion concerning the consumption of alcohol, there are only two rules to strictly adhere to. Never get behind the wheel of a car after having consumed alcohol—forget limits, the tolerance should be zero. Never get in a car whereby the driver has consumed alcohol. Your life is worth more than a free ride. Get the bus or pay for a taxi.

Secondly, never leave a friend unattended when you have been drinking. People do stupid things when drunk, never assume they can take care of themselves!

When attending a private house party:

- Don't feel pressured to drink just because everyone else is. You are your own person and it's possible to have fun *without* alcohol. Live according to your values.
- Only bring as much alcohol as you can safely and politely drink yourself. Two bottles is adequate, one (or less) for yourself, the other to share—but to

bring a case of wine is to invite disaster.

- Bring a bottle for the host, but do not expect them to crack it open at the party. This is usually considered a 'gesture' of re-stocking the cellar. Make it a nice bottle and suggest it is for the host's enjoyment at a later date.

- Do not arrive on an empty stomach. Unless you know a dinner party is planned, or at least had a hearty supper prior, make sure to line your stomach pre-drinks. Crisps and carrot sticks do little to help you when it's too late.

- Book a taxi in advance and stick to your planned exit time. Best you leave when you planned than to inconvenience your host in having to sort out a ride home for you or creating a makeshift bed.

- Respect the belongings and the home of your host. Skinny dipping in a well stocked Koi pond is never a good idea. Sliding down the stairs on heirloom silver trays is just as foolish, unless of course your host suggested it.

- Remember *every point* in what makes polite conversation. Just because you are drunk it doesn't make you amusing, intelligent, or worse, right about everything.

When drinking in public places, these codes of conduct should help you to remain dignified and assist you in having a good time:

- Don't feel pressured to drink alcohol just because everyone else is. You are your own person and it is possible to have fun without being 'merry'. Live your own values.

- Never accept a drink from a stranger. If asked to join someone for a drink under the guise of a 'date' make sure you witness the pouring or serving of your drink with your own eyes.

- Never leave your drink unattended or in the care of someone else, ever, anywhere. The seemingly 'classy' places attract undesirables too. Sexual predators and thieves won't help you out by wearing signs on their heads to identify themselves, and they aren't all dressed like vagrants either. Be suspicious, be cautious, be safe.

- The consumption of alcohol, unsociable behaviour and crime like to fraternise. Choose your drinking partners and establishments wisely. If you don't like the 'vibe' of a place, move on.

- The moment you or a member of your drinking party becomes, loud, aggressive, overly obnoxious, or threatening, it's time to leave. Don't wait until someone is throwing punches or punching in 999 on the telephone. Be one step ahead.

Be reliable

We all rely on somebody. Dependability is an attribute required of a good husband, wife, parent, and employee. There is simply no avoiding it. In order to be considered a good human being, your reliability and dependability will need to be honed to perfection.

From the beginning of time we relied on our parents or caretakers for our most basic of needs. It is a natural human desire to want intimate, reliable relationships that provide a sense of value and belonging. At the very core of it, we all hope that the people we are closest to are willing to put our feelings and needs ahead of other trivial things. We should all be able to rely on family, friends, partners, and the people we work with to 'do their bit' to help our lives run smoother. Doing life is a team effort.

Many people, namely the loners and melancholy, try to live their lives in a bubble, reliant only upon themselves and feel they don't need the help of others. Quite often they boast about the fact that they "don't need nobody" (poor English intended). Yet, they really do! Many people in fact; They rely on their bus or train driver to get them to work on time. They rely on someone in the sandwich shop to make their lunch. They might rely on a dog walker to keep their dogs happy, or a cleaner to keep their house in order. No man or woman is an island, we live in communities and we must communicate with people in order to live day to day. We must *trust* enough to rely on others, and be reliable ourselves.

Who might rely on you? Are you effective and helping to uphold your end of the bargain? Are you doing all you can to help someone's day run smoother? An unreliable person is someone who lives out their day selfishly when they see someone beside them struggling with something that they can easily help them with. It feels good to give, it feels good to be relied upon, and to serve. It gives you a sense of wellbeing and purpose.

It is an emotional hazard when you use this sense of being relied-upon for validation, however. It feels nice to be thanked for all you do and to be complimented on how reliable you are but when you are *only serving in order to receive this compliment* it undoes the honour your soul feels from serving *without expectation*. Refrain from offering more help than you can comfortably give, nor offer help for self-glorification. If you want to offer someone your help, then do so out of the goodness of your own heart and your desire to humbly serve them, not for the 'exchange' of compliments or glory.

People soon see through those who are constantly offering their 'help' when all they really want is to be made to feel important or to look good to an audience. Help behind the scenes, performed quietly and with humility means more than help given in the public eye. Do not give in order to be *seen* to be giving.

Ways to express and improve upon your reliability:

- Be a good keeper of time. There are very few good reasons to be late. Wear a watch, write your commitments down. Perform them at all costs.
- Manage your commitments. It is better to say you cannot help than to over commit yourself and disappoint others.
- Communication is king. We are all prone to flounder at some time or another, just don't 'surprise' someone with your failure. If you have to let someone down, let them know at the first opportunity. They have a greater chance of pulling in a favour from someone else or finishing the task themselves. You may not have completed your commitment on this occasion, but at least you were reliable enough to let them know.
- Let your actions rise above your excuses. Be clear on what you can achieve, and do all you can to make sure you keep your word. Your *actions* are what demonstrates reliability, not empty promises or poor excuses.

Loyalty

In modern first world society, the majority of people are living for themselves and for self-gratification rather than living to serve and love others. We live in an 'I' culture, not a 'we' culture which can seem quite normal, but only serves to break down relationship between people.

This is sad of course, but worry not about the loyalty of others in your life and care instead about yours, for you cannot control the way other people react to you, only your personal actions. When you lift yourself up to high and exacting standards, making sure to care about people and put them first, you set the best example.

Loyalty is only gained by people who are open and willing to love. You cannot expect loyalty from people if you mistreat them. You also cannot expect loyalty to last forever, so do away with the expectation that, 'because someone cared enough five years ago', they will feel the same way today. Trust and loyalty are built on a foundation of ongoing connection, so things may sour when you aren't consistently nourishing a relationship with someone.

Loyalty is something we exchange in loving, caring, nurturing and stable friendships and relationships. Instead of seeking loyalty from others you should be *earning* it every day.

People who demand respect and loyalty rather than obtaining it by default are putting themselves on a pedestal. The culture and reputation they are building around themselves demonstrates that they think so highly of themselves that others are not worthy unless they dance to their merry tune Be wary of these people as though they may expect *your* loyalty, they very rarely reciprocate.

Be loyal to your own heart, be loyal to your morality and be loving, gentle and caring to those around you. Be loyal to those that uphold this example too. Loyalty given to you will happen naturally if you set an example first.

Reputation by association

In England, though we hate to admit it, many of us are of the opinion that a person is defined by the company they keep. Why else would we be so keen for our children to associate with the right friends, or ourselves live in a 'good' street or town. It's better and far more comfortable for us to live our lives beside people who complement our values. We know what to expect of one another.

When you spend time with people who are thin on morality, manners and common decency, as if by osmosis, your reputation and self-worth will begin to fall inline with theirs. This is evidenced in generations of young people living in 'rough' areas. Good kids get swept up in gang culture, crime and immorality. The world is *telling* them they will have this identity because they see the 'gang' as a whole—they are seen as guilty by association. It may not be true, there are some very decent people living in these kinds of neighbourhoods yet because they entertain these 'bad' people socially, it appears they share the same principles.

Hard to move away from, granted, but there are ways in which you can safeguard yourself, your partner, and your children against destructive reputations and negative influences.

Never forget that your identity is *yours alone, to do with as you please.* Though we are not guilty by association, we are very much *exposed* to the influences around us, so why torture yourself? If you are surrounded by destructive thought patterns, behaviours and influences then you need to make a decision. Do you want to look guilty by association and expose yourself to the realities, and ultimately the temptations of this reputation? Or do you want to lead a better life which is inherently more positive in both thought and action?

This decision is available to everyone—young and old—who socialise with others who are mixed up in drinking, drugs, gang culture, sexual immorality, those with contempt for the rules of society, and people who have negative and destructive lifestyles. While we mustn't have contempt for these people, or judge them, we must *decide* if we should distance ourselves from the temptation of getting wrapped up in their ways.

Are the people you are spending your time with serving you and uplifting you? Are they honest, decent, honourable people, or are they tempting you into things that you know are bad for you? They may make you *feel* like you belong, but for whose benefit are you in a friendship with them? If you were to leave their company, will they still support you, or will they condemn you? If the answer is condemn you, then it sounds like you are there only to validate them and enable their bad behaviour. This is a one-sided friendship and one that is not healthy. This type of relationship is often seen in abusive relationships, gang culture, or a bully-victim scenario. When one person controls another in order to feel a sense of power or personal validation, it is a dangerous situation for both your physical and mental wellbeing.

Relationships and friendships are destructive when the time spent together is shrouded in drama, negative thinking and speaking badly of others, or if you are carrying out or witnessing destructive and sinful behaviour. Choose wisely who you spend your time with because despite what you know in your heart, you *will* look guilty by association and the time spent with those people will only serve to drag you down and perhaps tempt you in the long run.

A fine person should set an example, not ingratiate themselves in the lives of those who are living negative, destructive and immoral lifestyles, *unless they are there to help*. Be the light to these people but don't validate what they are doing by passively hanging around with them in order to make yourself or them feel better.

If you have spent enough time trying to lift negative associates out of the quagmire with no result, it's time to move on to pastures new. Not everyone is destined to lead a positive life, it has to be a personal choice that an individual makes in their journey. Don't let negative individuals persuade you to give up on your chance.

Watch your silent reputation signals

It is not only what you do and say and who you spend your time with that paints a picture of who you are, but also your 'silent' signals.

To name a few; rolling your eyes, making faces, turning your back on people, thinking you should have preference of a seat at a dinner table or in a queue, not opening doors or offering your help to someone who might need it.

The art of good etiquette is demonstrated in as much of what you *don't* do, as much as what you do. Turn frowns into smiles, keep negative thoughts to yourself, be open and pleasant to everyone you meet and have a sense of awareness of what you are doing at any given moment and how it can make those around you feel.

Be mindful of others, be mindful of the example you are setting and remember, that while the world may tell you that reputation doesn't matter, that you should be comfortable to live a selfish life—'YOLO', and to hell with the rules—your reputation *does* matter, a whole lot. At least, it should do if you want to be considered a lady or gentleman!

Sexuality

Sexuality, or moreover, sexual *immorality* is the ruthless killer of the good reputation. Poor public conduct when it comes to sexuality does very little in favour of the good reputation. This is a lesson for both genders and one that must be openly discussed when a young person is coming of age.

Despite what you may *feel* liberates you in your sexual conduct, it should be of no consequence to your peers or the public. What is experienced by you and known by others should be two very separate things.

Public attitude sadly, is more forgiving when it comes to men. We live in a culture that delights in and almost worships the male sexual reputation. Being somewhat of a 'lady-killer' is good. Men are encouraged to have sex, lots of it, and with as many women as possible. Meanwhile for women the opposite is true. We objectify and uphold the virgin, the demure wife, and though we live in a sexually liberated society that now openly talks about and 'sells' sex for women, we still call those women names if they actually do and act as we *say* they can. During this chapter we will remain careful to not argue on what is 'morally right', but there are certain things that can be learned from the viewpoint of common decency, etiquette, and reputation management. While sex is good, some public behaviour and attitudes surrounding it are not.

As humans, we *all* have, (or will have) our own sex life (full, or not), sexual appetites and urges. Yet many people seem to find it necessary to constantly talk about theirs, displaying and thrusting it all in other people's faces. Making love becomes less than lovely when you involve other people, and this includes talking about it! Sexual relationships should be treated as a sacred bond and something enjoyed in private. It is a time when two people are at their most intimate, and their most vulnerable. So when you treat this precious thing with disrespect by sharing your most intimate secrets, or worse, secrets of a partner (no matter how long or short term), you break that trust, and sully your reputation in the meantime. Not only will you be judged by the person whose secrets you shared, but by the person you shared them with. Times have changed. There *has* been a sexual liberation, but we don't all need to know about it! It *can* remain unsaid. We all have sex, that's a fact, but a boring one.

While in no position to judge individuals on their sex life and what goes on behind closed doors, people are well within their rights to judge your conduct and reputation surrounding that behaviour, **if it is out in the open**. What we witness or overhear, we have a right to feel uncomfortable about, if it makes us so.

So how do you manage a **public reputation** that is built upon this very natural thing to do? **We don't talk about it!** I know, I know, it's an odd thing to state given what generations who have 'gone before us' worked so hard to achieve, this sexual liberation. By all means indulge, but don't indulge the rest of us with the stories we don't want to hear.

This modern obsession with sex and talking about it has done little for people besides leading them down a slippery path of trading self-worth, obtaining sexually transmitted diseases, having to deal with unplanned pregnancies and racking up reputations. While at the moment you may not *think* you care about your reputation, someday you might. Your future husband or wife and in-laws might, and sexy-selfies, sex-tapes, and gossip may rear their ugly heads and come back to bite you in the bottom, long after you've settled into your relationships.

It's quite simply best not to talk about it to anyone other than the person you are most intimate with.

Sexual reputation management

Keep it confidential. Don't talk about sex in great detail to anyone other than the person you are intimate with. If you are concerned about a sexual intimacy and feel it is not right or you are being pressured or exploited then you *must* confide in a trusted friend or medical professional.

Don't spill the beans! It is absolutely no-one's business when you finally do have sex with a partner, how often, where, when and for how long. While you might get an immediate congratulations or have a little giggle over it, there stays a mental note in that person's mind of how many notches are on your bedpost. That information is yours and yours alone. How would you feel if you knew your significant other tells their friends intimate details of your relationship, including 'rating you' and letting them know what you are 'up for'? How would you feel if a one-night stand told all of their friends too? One of those very people might see you in a business meeting the next week, or could be a future in-law. It's just not cool to spill the beans. Gossip is harmful to the reputations of all involved.

Drink loosens lips. We all like to talk about odd and taboo things when we've had a few drinks. Our inhibitions are lost and we think it acceptable to tell our friends what happened during a sexual encounter. Hold your tongue! While everyone may laugh about it at the time, chances are they'll remember every detail of what you said the next day, and remember it for a long time. People are like magpies when it comes to shiny new gossip. The next time you and your partner are all drinking together with these friends it's highly likely the conversation (and sordid details) will come up again. *"Remember when you told us that Harry liked to do it in…"*. While the person may think it's funny relaying the story, Harry may not! Save yourself and your partner from the embarrassment and keep your private life exactly that, private.

Drink also loosens hips! Speaking of alcohol getting us talking, it also tricks us into thinking we are sexier than we really are. Dirty dancing and gyrating isn't particularly becoming in public places (save it for the bedroom), and while you may be the sweetest, most virginal person on earth, as soon as you start busting out your stripper moves on the dance floor (no matter how fabulously artistic or acrobatic they may be), you are essentially showing the dance floor what you can do in the bedroom (or think you can do). Dancing like that is 'encouraging' people to view you in a sexual way, even if that isn't *your* intention. Some forms and styles of dancing could be considered a mating ritual and attracts just as much unwanted attention as expected. Keep it clean, and save that side of you for the bedroom. Your great uncle Nigel doesn't want to see you dropping it like it's hot, nor should you want him to!

Keep the numbers low, or make out they are. People have a fascination with numbers. We like to keep score about everything, from what marks you got in a recent exam, to how much your house cost. We like numbers because it sorts us out, it grades us, separates the weak from the strong. We are highly competitive creatures and while we like to think that a high number of sexual partners will profess just how 'wanted' we are and how successful we've been at persuading people to go to bed with us, it actually just makes us look slutty and severely lacking in self-respect. Have you really found 'x' amount of people that you really wanted to get intimate with, or were they just a number to add to your collection to make you feel better about yourself—to increase your score?

So you ask, how many is *too* many?

Sadly there is no correct answer, while some people might think three is a nice modest number, to others it may be shocking. A lot of people think that ten partners is nothing, and they are in awe of their friend who can list over twenty-five partners. When you hear numbers over double digits, it's highly likely a lot of them were flings, one-night stands or worse, paid for, because the average real relationship usually lasts a while and 'good' girls and boys don't jump in the sack with a new beau right away. While your number may be way above that, the best thing to do is to **never share it.** People will make assumptions based on your number, whether it is high or low. They also like to spill the beans after a fall out, someone might casually mention how many people you've slept with in order to harm your reputation. Don't let them in on your business in the first place. That information is never truly safe.

Beaus minding their own business. Future spouses may also ask how many sexual partners you have had (if they know you are sexually active). You should decide for yourself what to do here as there are pitfalls to both being honest and telling white lies. Keeping to a modest number is always good if you absolutely must share, but remember, if you do have a reputation and are known to have been with some people, your partner can probably count for themselves after spending some time with you socially. It's always awkward turning up somewhere with a new beau and someone you've slept with is in the room. The atmosphere can be palpable, or the gossip mill can start and your beau will hear on the grapevine that you are 'known' to that other man. Which is not a good thing if you told him you only slept with one other man, a previous boyfriend who he already knows of! The absolute best answer you can give if he/she really insists on knowing is, "I've had a couple of serious boyfriends/girlfriends" then dig your heels in if they ask for more details. While they may be your current squeeze, there are some things you do have a right to keep to yourself. As for knowing the details about them, it's best not to ask. It's not *your* business either. If you have doubts about their sexual reputation and can't seem to trust them over it, or keep it in the past where it belongs, then ask yourself what you are doing with that person in the first place?

Intimate trust and blabbermouths. Sadly, a lot of people have experienced their reputations being damaged by partners who have blabbed about their encounters. This usually happens when the parties involved slept together on a one-night stand, or after a very short period of time. While not a nice scenario to have to face, it should have been somewhat expected because if you don't know them well enough to trust him not to talk, then you certainly shouldn't have trusted them enough to share your body. If you don't know someone well enough to know how they conduct themselves when it comes to intimacy and their respect of others, then stay away until you can be sure. The same goes for you and what you share. It is only decent to keep quiet about an encounter, no matter what you thought of it. If it pains you not to be able to share, then you need to evaluate why you are doing so. Those who gossip about their sexual experiences and partners are often seeking validation and approval, clearly in all the wrong places.

How to undo any of these misgivings, start now!

- Stop talking about sex with anyone other than your long term partner.
- Stop listening to other people when they gossip about sex—change the subject.
- Keep the past in the past, share only what you have to, when you have to.
- Be sober when the subject of sex is something you need to discuss with your partner.
- Act sexy for your partner only. It doesn't attract the right sort of attention in public.
- Don't make a big deal of your 'sexuality' publicly, especially not on social media. The people that do are probably being paid.
- Respect the people you have been intimate with and demand the same from them.
- Cut your losses from those who betray you intimately, this includes friends and partners.
- Wait, wait, wait and wait some more before entering into a sexual relationship.
- Never send text messages of a sexual nature or including graphic content.
- Stop the one-night stands, though you may be consistently sold the idea that one-night stands are fun, why is it called 'the walk of shame' the next day? They serve only to spread diseases and ruin your reputation.

While you may already have some interesting history when it comes to your sexual conduct, it isn't too late to start behaving well. Many of us 'have a past', but the difference between those who succeed in long-term intimate sexual relationships and those who do not is that those who 'get ahead' realise that being sexually explicit in their behaviour does nothing but build poor reputations. Destructive sexual attitudes can damage relationships both past, present, and future and do nothing but harm you emotionally in the long run.

If you continue to trade on your sexuality, people will begin only to see you in this light when in reality you have so much more to give. Who would want to date and treasure someone who still lives in that headspace? Really begin to see yourself and your intimacy as something to be won, respected and treasured and it will become so! If you keep giving it out for free to anyone who flashes you a winning smile, the value decreases significantly.

Allow second chances

If you or someone you know has 'had a past', it doesn't mean that they are still living out their lives practicing what earned the negative reputation in the first place. Of course, it is hard to forget the misdeeds of someone who stole from you, cheated on you, betrayed you or committed a crime but do you need to judge people based on their past all the time? Give people grace and the space to grow.

The world as a whole likes to hang onto the idea of guilt and that we must 'pay' for our wrongdoings, but there is a better way! It has been explained before that the very core meaning of etiquette is to make someone feel comfortable in your presence, so judging someone based on what you know about their past is keeping them stuck in that loop of negativity and isn't very gracious on your part.

How can we ever move on and learn to grow if we won't forgive the past and evolve into better people? If you want to have a better reputation, first you must learn to see others deserving of a fresh start too. When you think ugly thoughts about people, the mirror reflects that attitude and heavy judgement. You wear your thoughts on your face, so you need to be graceful towards others at all times.

In order to forget your own past and to forgive others you need only remember that we are all somewhat naive, prone to selfishness, often tempted by the world and all the bad choices it has to offer.

Be the light, the one who extends grace, forgiveness and kindness to all, you may never know when you need an ounce of that same grace in return.

Avoiding embarrassment for all

If this entire book could be condensed into one lesson, then this simple core value is the aim of everything you are being taught, the very essence of English Etiquette:

In every situation in life, you should do your utmost to make everyone feel comfortable.

This means minding your manners, standing up for what is right, taking the quiet, gentle and conservative approach, being considerate of and respecting all races, religions, cultures and feelings, and above everything always putting others before yourself.

There is no greater man or woman to walk this earth than the kind who love, nurture, encourage, protect and care about people.

SOCIAL GRACES

Common sense in communication

Common sense is the most crucial social grace of all. It is common sense not to step out into busy traffic, it is common sense to blow out a candle before you retire for the night but it is even more common sense to watch what you say to people. Stupid actions are stupid actions, we learn from those easily as the repercussions are almost always immediate. Cars knock us down and houses burn down but are you sure what you say will impact the person you are speaking to in a positive way? Will it portray you in a positive light?

It is common sense therefore not to gossip, to keep conversation light, to compliment rather than condemn and not to get too hot under the collar about any particular subject. We have a culture of celebrating the outspoken and the controversial conversationalist, sure, they may bring attention, but is it for the right reasons?

Save your overbearing opinions, your judgements and your condemnation. People don't like to hear it any more than you do.

Common sense in conversation should be extended to absolutely everyone. Who likes to be told they are wrong, or stupid, or their opinions don't matter or aren't as intellectual as yours? The finest conversationalist is the one who thinks before she speaks and if it won't serve the conversation in a polite, uplifting and dignified way, she won't say anything at all!

Right place, right time, right frame of mind

Are you living fully in the present of where you are right now, or are you living for the past or the future?

Before you venture out anywhere for the day, ask yourself, "Am I emotionally available and in a pleasant enough state of mind to honour those around me? Will my presence be a blessing to others or will my attitude lower the mood?"

Never accept an invitation to a party if you are feeling blue, never go out to the supermarket if you are feeling sour or bitter. Never invite a friend to tea just so you can bitch and complain about someone. This isn't to say that your feelings and emotions aren't valid, but is it necessary to subject an unsuspecting public to them? What can you do to lift your mood before you go out into the world? Can you sooth yourself with some prayer, meditation or listening to something uplifting? Should you get some sleep, or some rest for your soul?

Social graces count on you being a pleasant, fully functioning part of society, not a miserable bore who is intent on ruining things for everyone else. You know the girl, you see her at parties sitting in the corner bitching about what her boyfriend did, how her friend let her down, and how everything is terrible. Don't be her. Her energy is draining and people eventually tire of it.

Be in the right mood, at the right time, in the right place. Else, stay at home until you are feeling at peace about everything.

Eye contact

Eye contact says a lot about a person, we know we must look people in the eye when we are speaking to them, and when this doesn't happen we feel uneasy. Some people take this to the extreme however and gaze at you with too much intensity.

Make sure whenever you are speaking to someone directly to look them in the eye, but don't stare. It's ok to 'flick' your gaze to something else for a moment, perhaps to your teacup as you pick it up to take a sip, or towards a door as someone enters, but never let this last for more than a few seconds as it gives the impression you have left the conversation or are interested in things going on around you rather than the speaker. When you look at someone your eyes will naturally dart around the face, if you stare wide-eyed into theirs as though you are attempting to hypnotise them it may give your company 'danger' signals and put them off.

Always refrain from staring at something on a person that you find bewitching. This may be a bad wig, a scar or mole on their face or something else you'd be uncomfortable asking them about or addressing directly.

Saying the right thing

We all 'put our foot in it' sometimes. It's like we can't help ourselves but what we *can* help is learning to master good conversational skills. There are hundreds of ways in which you can master better conversation and speak confidently to anyone, but here are a few tried and tested quick-wins that will help you with the basics.

No one likes a sob story. Everyone has their own problems, so unless you know someone *very* well they aren't likely to want to help you out with your sob story about not being able to pay the bills, how you just got dumped, or that things are just rubbish for you at the moment. Of course, if you must share this information, make a joke out of it or share it in such a way that demonstrates that you aren't expecting the listener to either give you advice or fix the problem for you! "My flat got broken into last week, so annoying but at least they left the cat" is far more upbeat and emotionally removed than "My flat got broken into last week, they stole all my precious photo albums, I've been down in the dumps ever since and just can't sleep". Imagine some acquaintance saying these things to you. Which one are you able to respond to better? Think of the poor person you are speaking to and remember that sob stories are depressing.

Never speak about politics. Unless you are at a political convention or are in a debate team, politics is never a polite social conversation for ladies or gentlemen. Of course you can have political opinions or persuasions, but it is hard to evangelise people who have so very obviously made their minds up about political issues, as have you. No use in trying to get someone to switch camps if you aren't willing to either. Political conversations rarely end politely. Stay away.

Never speak about money. Some people have it, others don't, it's never a comfortable conversation and is pretty vulgar. If you need financial advice, go to people by all means, but forewarn them that you are seeking their advice before you meet up. Talking about how much you or your partner or parents earn, or how much something you own is worth is tasteless.

Gossip is entrapment. You know it when you hear it, and when you see it going down. Body language 'gets close', voices drop to a whisper. If you can, get away, if you can't then dare not repeat it and for goodness sake don't make a judgement about the subject discussed unless you know *both* sides of the story.

People love to talk about themselves. Talking about yourself incessantly is impolite and frankly boring. Only speak about yourself on the topics on which you have been asked. Always probe your companion to talk about what *they* like and what they think. It helps you to get to know people better and demonstrates that you are interested in them more than talking about yourself.

Mind your language. You might not care about using the S, F, or C words but your company might. Moreover you could be within earshot of other people and children. Mind your manners and mind your tongue! A person of class *never* swears or curses.

Never speak about other people in a negative light. You never know if who you are speaking to is associated with that person, and speaking of people in a bad light reflects poorly on you. Speak only positive things or nothing at all, even if your conversation partner begins to speak negatively about someone you may know. Hold your tongue and keep your ears open. You'll learn more about that person's character than who they are gossiping about.

Turn the volume down. Not everyone who shares public space with you wants to hear what you have to say, speak at an appropriate volume for your venue.

Correspondence and stationery

Correspondence is not what it used to be. What with emails, text messaging and Facebook we no longer have to wait for, nor learn how to craft socially acceptable messages. It seems politeness has fallen by the wayside, and with it decipherable language. While your friends may use Facebook to invite you to a party, be the difference and call them on the telephone to respond.

Nothing can replace good old pen and paper written in your own hand. If your handwriting is shocking, then pick up a course (there are plenty of them for free online) and practice until it is legible. We aren't all blessed with beautiful penmanship but we are blessed with the ability to make someone's day by sending them a thoughtful note via good, old-fashioned 'snail mail'.

Make sure to personally RSVP to every invitation instead of relying on your latest social media update to inform people of your whereabouts, and definitely don't offer messages of congratulations or condolences on social media to people you see in real life. Nothing speaks more about your regard for someone and better expresses your thanks or sentiments than a thoughtful and personal conversation, note or card.

Invest in stationery. In times past ladies and gentlemen were once well in supply of beautiful personalised stationery. There was a letter size and envelope for every occasion and etiquette so deeply ingrained in the proper way to handle and send it all. Though this practice has largely fallen out of fashion, it will serve you well to invest in some basic personal stationery to assist you socially.

Your shopping list should include:

Note cards and matching envelopes, ideally personalised. The note cards should be printed or engraved with your name, initials, or some form of identifiable mark atop. These are useful for sending thank you notes and casual correspondence. Many online retailers offer an 'off the peg' range as well as customised options depending on your budget, the prices can be very competitive.

Social cards. These are much like business cards but are casual in tone and include as little or as much personal information as you wish. They are useful for parties and handing out to friendly acquaintances (or potential love interests) with whom you have not met in a business setting. An example of the information to include could be as simple as your name and a contact email address or telephone number. Far classier than getting out your mobile phones or dashing about to find a pen in order to exchange details. If you are anxious about giving out too much information to all and sundry, include only your name and a contact email address, and if you wish you can always handwrite a telephone number in the remaining space. The conservative option is to include only your name and an email address. The person will have to make a greater effort to reach you, and forces them to think about what to write. Thus sorting the wheat from the chaff and less time wasted on your part. Especially useful in potential romantic situations as it is far more exciting to receive a thoughtful email detailing how lovely it was to meet you than a simple dry text. Who knows if you want that person to know your phone number right away anyway?

A good handwriting pen. If you don't own one, then it is time to invest. A good pen does more for your penmanship than you might realise and encourages you to write thoughtfully and at a slower pace. Invest in a nice pen for your beautiful new stationery and correspondence, you'll be glad you did.

There are plenty more options for personal stationery and far too many to list here, but the basics as listed above should take you places.

Texting is the enemy, the telephone is your friend

In years gone by, if we wanted to speak to our friends we used to call them up! To those of a certain generation, do you remember that? We spoke to our friends and love interests on the phone, sometimes for hours on end, sharing stories, laughing, giggling and building a personal bond. If we'd phone their home and they weren't there we might have a short conversation with their parents, friends or siblings, who we knew by name and who knew of us. We built relationships like this, but this practice has all but died. It's time to revive it.

Texting has replaced real connection creating a lonelier, colder, solitary existence. With our fast-paced social media concerned society we are used to consuming information fast. We now SnapChat or text our friends with gossip, information, or invitations and just sit and wait for their response. We have lost the pleasure of *conversation*, of waiting for them to be available for a nice chat and to give each other our full attention. "Wnt 2 meet 4 drinks?" has replaced a phone call where you could have asked the same thing and arranged a place and time, or made an alternative plan. We used to be able to hear the tone and inflection of one's voice and judge how someone felt, and ask them if they wanted to talk about it if we picked up on any sadness in their voice. Now we just accept a text of "Sry, busy" as verbatim and we go about our day. Relationships are built through listening, not reading.

Pick up the phone! Talk to people, hear the *life* in their voices. Warmly invite people to your dinner party or out for a drink. Pick up the phone and share congratulations, or let someone know you are thinking about them. Don't let a little screen dictate how you communicate.

Many of our contemporaries are now so used to this way of life they don't know what they are missing. Be the difference. Let people know that you expect them to call you with an invitation, or for a chat, and lead by example by doing exactly the same.

Relationships, both personal and professional are built on sound and sight, by hearing the tone and inflection of voice, hearing that special tone in the voice of someone who cares and has time to hear what you have to say. This communication and grace cannot be matched by a QWERTY keyboard, no matter how fancy the technology. "Hahaha" can never replace the sound of real spontaneous laughter. Stop missing out.

Entertaining and hosting

Some people love to throw parties and some people don't. If you are in the former camp then it is fair to say that you like spending time with people and are good at making people feel at ease in your company. This is great, but there are a few things that you should consider, whether you are used to hosting events and parties or not:

Environment. Is your house or the venue clean? Some never bat an eyelid at a bit of mess but other people can't see past it. I am one of those people, if someone has their husband's pants hanging about airing after being in the wash I can't help but zone in on that. A sense of decorum is not just meant for public, it should also extend into your home. Think to yourself, "Are any personal items on display that may make someone I am about to invite into my home feel uncomfortable?". It may be underwear or clothes lying about, perhaps your sanitary items are on full display in your bathroom, or you've got bank statements piled on the kitchen counter. Your house needn't be spic and span if you aren't that way inclined, but at least try to have enough sense to remove any potentially embarrassing or shocking items from view of your guests.

Are you accommodating enough? Have you catered for the vegetarian, for the recovering alcoholic, or the pregnant lady who can't eat seafood? Don't put on a party just for the majority, think about the individual needs of every person attending. If you've suggested children come too, have you thought about how they will be entertained, fed, and left to sleep if they need to?

Overnight guests. If you invite people to stay overnight, then the kindest thing to do is offer them your most comfortable place to sleep. If they refuse then offer them a place to get some privacy to change or shower rather than just expecting them to 'get on with it'. I've lost count of the amount of times I've been 'offered' a place to stay when in reality it is a sofa without even so much as a blanket. If you offer to host someone, for hours or a full weekend, make them feel as comfortable as possible and in no way a burden to you.

Being a polite guest

It's just as crucial to learn how to be a good guest as it is a host. We all have funny little quirks and nuances but we needn't subject everyone to them.

If you have been invited to dinner, ask if the host would like you to bring anything. If the answer is no, then don't insist but instead take a token gift. Chocolates, flowers or a small gift like a scented candle or gourmet food item are usually well received.

Many like to take a bottle of wine to a party. If you do this, unless you know the host won't be offended, then let them know it is a gift just for them and set it aside from the rest of the dinner/drinks. It is bad etiquette to take a bottle of wine to a party and proceed to drink it yourself. It insinuates that the wine your host provided isn't good enough. Of course, if it has been specified to bring a bottle, then do so, but don't drink more than your share!

Think about your feet. Will you need to take your shoes off when you enter someone's home? Wear appropriate shoes that won't make your feet smell, take socks if you must and manicure your feet if you'll be barefoot. Don't wear ridiculous pin thin high heels to a dinner party, for whose benefit are those? Not the host's hardwood floors, that's for sure.

If you are staying overnight, enquire about what you need to bring and make sure you do. Also take appropriate nightwear (nothing too revealing), plus your own toiletries. Ladies never sleep on your host's pillow without first removing your make up. Get up at an appropriate hour in the morning and dress as soon as possible. Don't overstay your welcome and don't refuse breakfast or a cup of coffee if it is offered.

Watch the amount of alcohol you consume. Not only might you make a fool of yourself, but stumbling about in someone's home and vomiting into the pot-plants is a social faux pas difficult to recover from.

If you break it, you replace it—no arguments.

Offer to help clean and tidy, but don't argue if the host says no.

Write a thank you note within forty-eight hours and post it immediately, whether it was just for dinner or you stayed with your host for an entire week. Texting and emailing does not count. If you become very close with someone and see them often, then you may refrain from writing formal thank you notes as it becomes a bit much to send them so frequently. Express your thanks verbally with those closest to you. However on special occasions, such as an invitation to Christmas, a formal thank you still says a lot.

Eating in public

A lady or gentleman never eats in public unless they are *dining*. Fast food and eating in the street is not considered dining, and is never attractive. Eating at a desk is also not the best way to spend time on what is supposed to be a break from your work.

When eating at a private home or restaurant, be it a fast food chain or a fancier place, there are a few things that you must consider regardless of your surroundings, or your company:

- Use a napkin, place it on your lap when you are eating and use it to dab the corners of your mouth. Dripping sauce and food remnants on your face is never attractive. Napkins are there for a reason, use them.
- Never chew with your mouth open, nor speak with your mouth full. This is

something we are all taught as children, yet many adults still forget to practice this simple rule.

- Serve others before yourself. He or she who dives in first is not only a glutton, but also rather selfish.
- If you need to use the loo, do so before you sit down to order. Being left alone to eat while your company goes off to do their business in the middle of the main course is never fun. If you find yourself needing the loo during a meal, at least wait until the main course is over and pay that visit before pudding.
- Don't drink too much alcohol, the reasons are obvious.
- If you are a picky eater or have allergies, discuss these with your waiter quietly. Your fellow diners need not hear about how asparagus plays up your IBS, or how you come out in hives if there is pepper on your plate.
- Elbows off the table and always sit up straight.
- Your bread plate is to your left, and your drinking vessels are to your right.
- Your fork should be held in your left hand and your knife in your right. Don't hold your knife like a pen, nor lick it or eat off of it. For goodness sake, never lick it!
- Compliment the staff on the food when deserved, and if you must complain do so quietly and with class.
- Thank your fellow diners for their company. If they have paid, thank them for their generosity.
- If you are eating in someone's home, be mindful that they have to clean up whatever mess you make. Offer to help carry plates to the kitchen (never stack them unless asked to do so, it may be expensive china), pour drinks, or do the washing up. Likely your offer will be declined, but what matters is that you offered.
- If you are eating in your own home, remember to compliment and thank your spouse, your friend or family member or whoever has fed you.
- Observe and be respectful of any prayer or thanksgiving someone may wish to say over the occasion.
- Follow up with a thank you note or review. If you have been particularly struck with your experience at an independent restaurant, share your positive experiences online via a review website, or recommend them to friends. Food feeds the body, but kind words nourish the soul.

Walking down the street

You'd be surprised at how frustrating it can be performing the simple task of walking down the street. People either walking too close, take up too much space, cut you up, stop dead in front of you, collide with you, or just plain get in the way.

Much like traffic, everyone should recognise which 'lane' they are travelling in and stick to it. If you like to amble, be aware that there may be people who want to walk faster than you, so walk slowly in a definite path, ideally a straight one. Those who are walking fast will judge the direction you are moving in and plan their overtake accordingly. Don't surprise them by suddenly pulling out into the fast lane.

The rule applies for making manoeuvres. You may want to cross the footpath and enter a shop, but make your signal and intention known *before* you move. Look around and into your blind spot. Some unsuspecting person could be coming up alongside you and unless they see you looking, they'll walk right into you.

If you are a wheelchair user or pushing a buggy, then of course you will naturally be given right of way in many circumstances, but that doesn't mean you should take advantage of this kindness and take up more space than you should.

Some people like to think they own the footpath and feel that you should be the one to get out of their way. These people have rotten attitudes. Many a time I have been 'hit' with a forearm of someone who didn't move just that few inches to meet me (or avoid me) half way. If that person apologises for colliding with you, apologise right back with a smile and say it's ok. If they don't, then you'll probably want to shout at them and glare, or make an example of them, but don't. It won't get you anywhere, it's unlikely they'll learn a lesson from it if they are rude enough not to apologise. The same goes for people who you step aside for, or open doors for in public places not thanking you. Just remind yourself that you are the **example**, and making a show or a mockery of them in public will undo all of the good work your example was setting.

Be the exception on the streets, not the rule.

Driving and road rage

What use is it getting angry behind the wheel of a car? Sure, people drive badly. They make mistakes and those mistakes can frighten you, but is sitting there waving your arms about and shouting expletives at the top of your voice really going to make all that much difference? Question this, if someone cuts you up with their trolley in a supermarket do you slam your breaks on, throw your arms up in the air, make noises like a horn and start swearing at them for their manoeuvre, whether intended or not? Thought not.

Swallow the hard truth, you aren't the world's best driver, and neither are ninety-nine percent of the driving community. The best and most considerate drivers on the road are actually driving instructors and their pupils, who follow the rules diligently. But my goodness how *those* drivers annoy us.

When you feel yourself bubbling up with rage, consider what is happening in the mind of the driver who cut you up. Grace is your best weapon, not car horns and rude gesturing.

Car windows are made of glass, and as much as people can see you picking your nose at a red light, they can also plainly observe your terrible roadside etiquette when you let rage take hold of you.

Keep your emotions in check behind the wheel! Not allowing things to fluster you may just save your life and someone else's. Driving erratically due to charged emotions is neither polite, nor clever.

Parking

Some of us are good at it, others not so much. Aside from going back to driving school there are a few parking etiquette observations to live by that make motoring a little easier on us all.

Do not park where you aren't supposed to, you'd be surprised about how many people do this.

Never park in a disabled space unless you have an authorised badge. Any person who violates these rules deserves a fine.

The same goes for parking in 'mother & baby' spaces. Don't park in them if you have no child in your vehicle (and your empty child seat isn't fooling anyone). Trust me, there are mothers who sit and wait for a space and will curse you when you get back to your car and drive away without a child in sight.

Never park across driveways, double park or block someone in, no matter how desperate you are for a space. Should you have to for a life-threatening emergency then leave a note explaining the event, but still be expected to receive a reprimand. Nothing angers people more than inconsiderate motorists.

The British queuing system

Oh the most glorious invention of civilised English society, a queue. Queues give everyone a fair chance, bring order to chaos and a sense of decorum to an otherwise painful and boring situation. With that in mind, the utmost attention should be considered to decorum and a sense of fairness. So this means no chewing gum, talking loudly, huffing, puffing, smoking, invading personal space, or other such unpleasantries.

By nature, the Englishman when put in close proximity with people they don't know, like to pretend the situation isn't happening, so it's "eyes forward, no eye contact and concentrate on the task at hand". Queuing is a very regimental and stoic event, and our behaviour should match accordingly. The people surrounding you deserve respect. When waiting for a long time, feel free to exchange pleasantries rather than making miserable discussion. "Well, at least we have some lovely weather while we are waiting" is far more pleasant than "How long have you been waiting for, they are so slow here it's unbelievable". Let someone else be the doomsayer in the queue. Never let on that you are tired, frustrated, bored or annoyed. Queues are quick to release inconsiderate behaviour in people. Keep your manners in line, as well as yourself.

It is highly likely that during the hours spent queuing over the course of your lifetime you will be met with queue jumpers, or those who have no regard for fairness. To reprimand a jumper, a simple "Excuse me, I do believe this gentleman was before you" should suffice. All other queuers will be in agreement. The offender will be made aware his bad manners have been noticed and will not be tolerated.

It is kind to let another person go ahead of you if you see that they are elderly, unwell or have small children who are becoming impatient. Let them know you are happy for them to go ahead of you but only offer this to a person immediately behind you. It makes no difference to the waiting time of the person directly behind them and displays kindness that may be matched by others in the line. Sometimes people need reminding of how good it feels to be charitable and offer other people priority over you.

Gum chewing

If you must do it, it should be reserved for dental benefit only. Chew only after a meal and for no more than five or ten minutes. Gum chewing for leisure or pleasure is frankly, grotesque, and need it be mentioned that spitting it out on the floor, or playing with your gum is déclassé. Chewing gum contains terrifying ingredients which you can find out for yourself if you are willing to do your research. Absorbing these ingredients into your bloodstream is bad for your health, and gum is a plastic. It will *never* biodegrade, essentially adding to our already overwhelming global pollution issues. Choose breath mints, or a breath spray as a kinder alternative overall.

Personal appointments

When you book a personal appointment make a note of the date and time somewhere reliable and keep to it! If you know you must break or rearrange an appointment then call to inform the organisation as soon as possible. Many of them are relying on your time-slot and business in order to put food on the table. Your missed medical appointment could have been better utilised to help someone who is very sick. Failing to turn up to an appointment is the height of rudeness. You should also call as soon as you know you are going to be late to *any* appointment, regardless of whether it is a personal or professional one.

Time is precious to people and you should respect it.

Demand the same from others. If your friend is consistently late, ask them to inform you next time if they will be running late. If you don't ask you don't get, some people simply need telling, but gently, of course.

Shopping

Sales assistants, a breed unto their own. In England we try to get as far away from them as possible and have an arsenal of quick responses, whether honest or not, to their incessant questions. Assistants in shops, be it a garden centre, cafe or a clothes store still *need* human interaction to make them feel useful. I have worked in retail and it is a misconception that sales assistants are there to annoy. Standing around all day surrounded by the same stock for a season soon becomes rather tedious when customers wave you off every time you ask if they need help.

The best salesperson is always the one who really listens to you and makes you feel valued, and you should be just as gracious towards them. They (hopefully) have in-depth knowledge of the item you are looking to purchase and you should be appreciative of that. Allow them to exercise their people skills. If we all did that, then sales forces overall would be a little less irritating.

Remember too that the future alternative to the plucky sales assistant is *self-service by way of robot*. Horror of horrors, who wants that?

If you have the time, and are just browsing there are many ways that you can make your sales assistant's day and get superior service while you are at it. Once you make a consistently good impression, upon every return to the store the staff will warmly welcome you back. It's a great feeling when you walk into a store and people know you by name and what you like. Whether that be cake, shotgun cartridges, or cardigans.

If you want to feel really valued, then make friends with them. It works very well in boutique and independent stores. Shops with a higher turnover of staff are harder to crack, but do try anyway. Retail staff move on quickly but once they remember your face, they'll treat you well wherever they work.

Shop with good manners. As soon as you walk in and smile at the staff, greet them with a sunny "Good morning/afternoon". Make sure to make good eye contact and strike up a conversation with a little statement about the day. "It's gloriously sunny out, I bet you can't wait to enjoy it", or "Blimey, it's busy in town today, have you been rushed off your feet?" They will of course reply (to which you acknowledge the response), and then it is likely they ask if you need any assistance (particularly true of clothing stores). If you are just browsing just reply kindly with "I'm just browsing today thank you", but for goodness sake, if you *are* looking for something specific tell them! They can then lead you right to the product and you have made them feel useful in the process. They are there to help you and what job satisfaction will they get if they are made to feel useless? It always pays to compliment the member of staff if they are wearing something nice from the store, compliments go a long way.

When you are looking for a specific product, rather than ask the staff member to show you where it is, ask for their opinion too. "I'm looking for a shift dress for work, do you have anything in a pink, or a spring colour?" This opens up the conversation far better than "Can you show me where your shift dresses are"? If they don't have any then talk around the subject, ask if they think they'll be getting any in, or what they think might suit you as an alternative to buy. It is *these moments* that add up to a nice day for all. Speaking to people and exchanging sunny conversation are what make the civilised world go round.

Just because you are talking to a member of staff doesn't mean you are under any extra pressure to purchase something.

Thank the member of staff for helping you. Be gracious and kind to everyone in the store. I often make sure to compliment other shoppers on a choice they have made, or in the fitting room if something looks particularly lovely. You never know quite who you'll meet and doing so puts a spring in everyones step. Shopping can be a wonderful social event and a pleasurable self-care experience rather than a chore if you have the correct attitude about it.

The simplest rules of social graces:

- Always say please. It costs nothing.
- Always say thank you. Thank everyone for everything, for the biggest things and the smallest of things. Thank them in words, gestures, written notes, gifts and compliments.
- Always say excuse me. Whether you need to leave a table, leave a conversation, ask someone to move out of your way, be pardoned for a burp, or need someone to repeat what they said. Excuse me is the politest of expressions after please and thank you.
- Ask permission. Whether to do something when you are under someone's roof, need to do something 'out of the norm' for the social situation (like take a phone call), or to borrow someone else's property.
- Say hello and goodbye. Even if you think you won't be noticed or missed. Company will remember your rudeness for not greeting them or saying farewell.
- Ask if you can help. Even if your offer is declined, it's the offer of sacrifice that will be remembered. A lack of assistance reflects poorly on you.
- Eat and chew properly. It's what sets us apart from the animal kingdom and demonstrates our sophistication and refinement. Don't let the side down or subject anyone to your mastication.
- Watch your words. Always speak words of kindness and encouragement. If you find you are in a situation where you can't even muster that, then keep your mouth shut! Words have the power to build people up, and they have the power to destroy. Speak ill of no one, even your greatest enemy.
- Knock on closed doors. Unless you own what is behind that door, if you are met with a closed door knock and wait to be invited to enter. Not only is it rude to just walk in, you might not want to see what is going on behind it. Some things you can't unsee.
- Give up your seat to the elderly, the infirm, and the pregnant. They need it more than you.

While we might not all be highly educated graduates, talented and highly regarded by others based on our achievements. Nor rich, successful, beautiful or famous, we can *all* be socially and emotionally intelligent if we but try.

It doesn't matter what your face looks like, what your CV says about you, or even your social or economic background, what matters most is how you show respect and treat other people. Remember social graces, be kind and considerate and above all show your appreciation for your fellow brothers and sisters in this beautiful, complex world.

Self-Control

Self-control in an out-of-control culture

Having goals and ambitions is fantastic, but how do you go about navigating life well in order to achieve them? Despite what you choose to do, you will have to deal with people every step of the way. Learning how to respect yourself and others in the process may take a lot of sacrifice of self and a great deal of control, because not everyone will be 'easy' to deal with. This is the very art of etiquette; knowing what not to do and say, before learning what to do and say.

People by design are passionate and opinionated, which is a wonderful thing when communicated correctly, but we often undermine ourselves by acting this way all the time, especially when we are feeling a bit negative. Not everyone wants to hear your opinion *all the time*, especially when it serves no purpose other than to bring people or a situation down. One must learn self-control and how to exercise it at all times for the common good of both yourself, and social harmony.

There are many things that may cause us to lose self-control. Physical loss of self-control can be brought on by our own means, for instance the misuse of alcohol or substances. It can also happen when we lose control of our poise and allow an issue to make us 'act out' physically or verbally. This can be evident in the use of negative and poor body language to show displeasure to a certain situation. Violence of course is the greatest physical manifestation of a lack of self-control, but every single one of these poise-shatterers can be controlled with the *mind*. Remind yourself of the importance of poise and consider what you can do to make an informed, mature decision about what to do, rather than reacting poorly in the moment and regretting it later.

This isn't to say you shouldn't *feel*, or live, or have fun, or be passionate, but it does require you to at least measure the situation and make a sensible decision about how you *want* to act before you leap.

Before you speak and before you react

While physical bodies are things that we must learn to control, our mind and emotions are the greater battleground. We have a whole world of emotion and experience going on inside of us, an entirely individual spirit with passions, opinions, likes and dislikes, love, hope, fear, anxieties and expectations. It's great to be in touch with our feelings, but we must learn to control most of them in order to be good and decent people. We must learn and exercise a sense of dignity, courtesy and propriety at all times, otherwise society would be a hot bed of emotion with tempers flaring, harmful experiences and odd encounters happening at every turn. You only need to walk through a busy town late at night to see people living out this existence—the ones who have had a bit too much to drink. Drunkenness reveals supercharged emotions or 'triggers'; bullying, arguments, sexual frustration, family issues, domestic problems and anxiety all have the same negative effect. They make you lose your poise and dignity.

Drunks lose their poise, speak what is on their mind (good and bad), act up, cause fights, abuse people (physically and verbally), cry, and bring up topics they wouldn't dare talk about when sober. The inebriated think they are invincible and in control of themselves (when they are clearly not) and worst of all, think there will be no consequences to their indecent behaviour.

We all need self-control in order to operate as a well rounded society. A sense of common decency, a code of conduct and pattern of behaviour that is expected from all of us. It is your *duty* to play your part.

What follows are a variety of very common triggers that may present a challenge to your sense of self-control. Included are some suggestions and guidance as to how you can act accordingly in order to keep your mind in the right place when faced with these challenges. Be the exception, not the rule.

Learning to forgive

It is a fact of life that one person or another may disappoint you at some point, and a few may even really hurt you. Still, an unforgiving heart is a woeful thing. Being able to forgive is one of the most graceful and kind things you can do. Holding onto grudges and treating people with the contempt you feel for them only reflects poorly on you, it isn't healthy to hang on to all that negative emotion.

Imagine this situation; you are at a party and spot a person in the room who did something to really hurt you a few years ago. You have not spoken to this person since and the relationship between you both is sour. They never apologised, and you haven't forgiven. Do you think that other people will be able to tell there is bad blood between you both? People can read emotion in an instant. Your whole body language and demeanour will change when you look at this person and your facial expression becomes filled with pain, anguish, hate, confusion, dislike and all the nasty feelings and thoughts you are having about that person.

The person you cannot forgive may feel two things in this situation. They may feel remorse, guilt, embarrassment, and shame—yet you look at them like you want to string them up and let everyone in on their dirty little secret. They feel like the whole room has eyes on them. That you might 'erupt' at any moment and cause a scene. Alternatively, they meet you with equal hate and bitterness. The party atmosphere will be ruined and you will no doubt make the time awkward for all those around you.

Who is the right person in this situation?

Neither of you, **forgiveness is a gift you give yourself**. It allows you to move on and rise above a situation, not to wallow in the past or continue to cause yourself anguish over the wrongdoings of another person.

Forgiveness isn't easy, but it is certainly easier to forgive than to forget. There are many ways that you can forgive both in heart and mind and things you can do or say that will express this release of negative energy.

How to forgive

Are you acting out of truth, or on behalf of someone else? So many people act out of false information and make judgements about others based on what a gossip *said* to them. Is your lack of forgiveness based on a situation of truth, or an assumption? Have you judged the person fairly based on a falsehood? When you only have half truths, or are 'hating' someone who did something indirectly (meaning they have an issue with someone else, but you have taken up the baton of judgement on their behalf), it shows you to be unfair, a gossip, and willing to be manipulated into passions that aren't your own.

Put the situation into perspective. Realise that the person may not have been thinking when they hurt you, or hadn't meant to. Perhaps they aren't as sensitive as you are. Perhaps they acted out of fear, or frustration or anger. You may not have deserved what happened or what was said, but does it really matter in the bigger picture? Think about whether you have all of your facts straight, is it really worth the bother to hold on to resentment? Some people like drama for the sake of drama, don't be one of them. Gain whatever perspective on the situation you can muster and act accordingly.

You can't fix everyone. This person may have done something to hurt you that they are continually doing to others. Clearly they have issues with their attitude, self-esteem and the way in which they view the world. Though you've probably spent hours deliberating over the right thing to say to make them realise that they have caused you pain, or to get them to see your point of view—it is highly unlikely to work as most humans don't like being told they are wrong. Some people get defensive and angry when they feel threatened or judged over their behaviour. It isn't your job to fix them. By all means, you can tell them they hurt your feelings but don't expect it to change them.

Stop expecting apologies. We all grew up being told to say sorry, but now as adults we live in a world of broken moral law and people like to make up their own minds about what is acceptable to say, and how one should act towards fellow human beings. There is no law to say we should apologise, the only thing that can spur us into doing that is our own conscience. It's a romantic and unrealistic ideal that everyone is expected to apologise. Learn not to *expect* apologies and you'll never be disappointed. That being said, make sure **you** always apologise.

Apologies are always appropriate. Even when you think you have done nothing wrong, you should always apologise because there is *always* something to apologise for. Despite being steadfast in your opinions or actions (right, or wrong) you can always apologise *for* the situation. Express remorse that you are in a disagreement. Apologise that they feel sad, or hurt, or confused. Apologise that your disagreement has even happened. Be apologetic for the awkwardness and confusion.

Set that caged beast free. Forgiveness doesn't always require communication, or relationship. It's ok to forgive without having to speak to the person you are forgiving. Often we feel like if we make the decision to forgive someone we give them a free pass to enter back into our lives again, and that we'll have to be friends with them—not so. Whether you let them back into your life, or even let them know you've forgiven them is entirely up to you. You only need to communicate that decision to your heart and your mind. You'll know the right thing to do when you forgive someone. Whether you should open up communication with them in order to release them from the bondage of your negativity, or just to silently release them back into the world again. When you have forgiven someone, you release the negative energy you felt towards them from your body and you will feel a sense of ease when in their presence or thinking about them. This isn't to say that you can allow them to mistreat you again, that you should forget, or even have them *in* your life. The forgiveness is for *you* firstly. Author Malachy McCourt wrote,

"Not forgiving someone is like drinking poison and hoping your enemy will die". Rather an unproductive attitude to have, no?

See the bigger picture. Remember, *you* have to live with the decisions *you* make. People will come and go in your life, they are there to enrich your life whether it be a positive or negative experience. Positive experiences give you joy, and negative experiences help you to grow and develop, to explore your conscience, personal standards and how you relate to the world. They help you learn lessons from the experience and use that knowledge to better navigate your relationships with the people in your future. It is all about perspective. Be thankful for the experience, no matter how much it hurt and realise that the person who caused you pain will live with the experience too. They might go on feeling remorse or regret forever, or they might grow through it just like you did and move on positively (whether they apologised to you or not).

Perfection doesn't exist. None of us are perfect and we all need forgiveness at some stage in our lives. It hurts when we truly want forgiveness, only to have that door shut in our face. It isn't a graceful way to live and it certainly isn't very loving. Don't harbor an ugly heart that lacks in compassion, understanding and perspective.

Hate and anger weighs heavy on the heart. You deserve better than to carry that heavy load for the rest of your life.

A proper relationship with alcohol

Nothing good comes from the abuse and misuse of alcohol. Any decent person knows that having 'one too many' is neither good for your dignity, overall health, or for the wellbeing of your family. We all know that when people drink too much they lose their inhibitions. What comes in its place is never socially edited and people often find themselves saying and doing stupid things that they wouldn't dare to when sober and aware of their faculties.

Do you really want to be the friend known to run off at the mouth, or the one who loses all self-control and dignity whenever you have too much to drink? I know there will be plenty of people who will launch a battlecry at the suggestion of reducing your alcohol intake. "It's fun to have a drink", thousands cry. Of course it can be fun to imbibe but you cannot deny it is seldom attractive when one goes overboard, and is usually followed with a period of regret. Regret for the things said and the potential repercussions to relationships especially.

Have you ever witnessed a gaggle of women who've had too much to drink?

Or felt threatened by an overbearing group of male louts? Not pretty or fun, is it?

Of course, alcohol is nice to enjoy in moderation. Why else would we have booming wine industries, independent craft beer companies and distilleries making lovely varieties of gins, spirits and whiskies. Yet where this pleasure falls down is when we *abuse* it. You only need look at our present day drinking culture with a critical eye to see just how terrible it is. Our bodies simply aren't designed to process alcohol and while we can handle a glass or two, the absolute soaking most people's bodies get on a weekly basis is causing widespread physical, financial and emotional harm.

So how can you enjoy alcohol safely, have a good time *and* keep your dignity? The secret is a double-pronged attack using two weapons. Respect for yourself and respect for alcohol. Respect for the product that it is, what it can do for us, and what it is capable of *doing to us*.

Drink moderately, and infrequently. Of course, this one seems like the easy answer but there are many reasons why we should drink moderately. Not only does it mean we won't abuse alcohol by consuming too much of it, we give ourselves a break from having to process it.

Our bodies where not designed to process heavily manufactured food and drink products. While we may see a grapevine in nature, we don't see a 'wine vine'. Our bodies are organic living things that are adept at processing things in their natural state, not the products of *altered* states of organic produce. Alcohol is incredibly acidic, and our blood is finely tuned to work at an optimum PH level of 7.4, which is slightly alkaline. Our stomachs are acidic at 1.5-3.5 on the PH scale. Every other organ in between has its own optimal PH scale. Imagine what all that alcohol is doing to your body when you go over the top. You are essentially undoing the fine balance of your bloodstream, as well as the PH of other organs, putting your body under incredible strain to re-balance itself.

Speaking of bloodstreams, your body is made up of an average of sixty percent water, so when you consume alcoholic fluids you are flooding your body with poison that it doesn't require. While we may be able to handle a glass or two (like dropping a glass of wine into a swimming pool of fresh water), it really struggles when the intake of alcohol is *replacing* your hydration and depleting your body of its life-force.

Alcohol also alters the mind, and while it sometimes feels good, it is also a great threat to us in many ways. Alcohol affects the nerves that pass messages around the body by slowing them down. The more you drink the *greater* the effect. The reason people often get more 'lively and fun' when they've had a drink is because alcohol specifically affects the part of the brain responsible for self-control. Your reactions also slow down considerably making you uncoordinated and slurring your speech. What your brain wants you to do and what your body does becomes separated. We can also experience a string of emotional responses. Some become aggressive, tearful or very depressed, and judgement becomes impaired. You may do things out of the norm like starting fights, dancing inappropriately or even going home with strangers, which is extremely dangerous.

The ground rules for drinking politely

Wear modest clothing. Gentlemen rarely marry women who dress inappropriately and women never find the shirtless man in the street even slightly arousing. The chances of an encounter with a drunk person who dresses inappropriately turning into a real romance are slim, especially if the first thing on your mind when you met was purely sex. If you wouldn't be happy to meet a new beau's parents, or be in the company of colleagues in the outfit you are wearing, then it's not appropriate for any occasion, *especially* when going out drinking.

Act and talk modestly. Don't engage in risqué conversation or act ridiculously. Unless you've had *a lot* to drink you'll find this uncomfortable anyway. These types of conversations are not spoken about so openly in daily life, so why engage in them now? Especially in public places with goodness knows who listening in? If you wouldn't talk to your friends about sex over a cup of tea and a biscuit, why are you doing it over a glass of wine? The same goes for the way you act. If you wouldn't usually gyrate against telegraph poles or 'sexy dance' on your local pub's table while sober, then please refrain. Groping is *never* appropriate.

Just be modest! While it doesn't guarantee you will avoid the attention of someone with bad intentions, it is more likely you won't be *directly* in sight if you act with dignity. The foolish drunk girl dressed like a tart and flirting with every man she sees is giving out a signal (intended or not) that she is 'available for the taking'. When alcohol is involved, neither she, nor the man with the 'intentions' are capable of making a correct judgement about one another, or what the other wants from them. Don't put yourself directly in the line of fire. Alcohol and subsequent immodest behaviour have the potential of fuelling sexual encounters which can be a point of regret for all parties—often with sad and sometimes life changing consequences. You neither want to be the person finding yourself in a situation you can't control, or the person accused of instigating unwanted affection or physical contact.

Question this: why is it that you don't think about outrageously flirting with and erotically dancing in front of men to get their attention and make you feel desirable in broad daylight after a couple of lattes with the girls, yet you'll happily do it twelve hours later after a few drinks? Too much drink makes you act stupidly and you lose class and dignity. There's no argument there, modest is hottest. Men, the same goes for you, good humour and conversation is so very attractive! Groping, staring at, drooling over and complementing a girl on her figure, telling her how sexy she looks and asking her to ditch her friends and come back to yours is *not* gentlemanly behaviour.

Plan your evening before you head out. These plans must include where you are going! Whether you are in your local town or a new place entirely, at least have some sort of idea of where you are going and with who. Heading out the door simply to get drunk at any watering hole or boozy establishment is throughly unbecoming. Also plan your transport both to and from your destination, book a taxi for a suitable time, there should be no reason why the dignified should be out after midnight. Always make sure you book or take a taxi rather than walking home if you are alone. When taking a taxi, make sure it is licensed and ideally travel with a friend to one singular destination.

A note for ladies: When going out for the evening with a female friend, invite her to stay with you or ask if you can stay the night at her house. Single girls travelling alone at night either in taxis or on foot are always at risk. We know this. Let someone know of your plans, where you are going, who with, and when you should be expected home. Honour your parents with this information, your flatmates, your boyfriend or husband, or even a friend on the phone. Just make sure *someone* knows your whereabouts. On occasions where alcohol is involved you should be *especially* vigilant.

Only by the night. Day drinking is rarely a good idea if you plan on having more than one. 'Normal' life is happening for most people and those stumbling around drunk will swiftly find themselves a nuisance. Alcohol dehydrates. Couple that with sitting in the sun in excessive daytime heat and you've got a recipe for lightheaded disaster. Day drinking should be reserved for special and formal occasions only such as a glass of Champagne to toast a wedding, or a Pimms on the lawn at a summer garden party. BBQ's in private homes and while on holiday are also acceptable places to have a drink in the day, but do refrain from sitting at a bar on a random Tuesday lunchtime sinking the Chablis like your life depended on it.

Drink safely. This means many things, drink moderately of course and don't mix your drinks, swapping between beer and wine and/or spirits. Also make sure you keep hold of your drink at all times. Unfortunately the act of spiking drinks is common. This is when someone adds a type of sedation drug to your drink without your knowledge. Some people do it 'for a laugh', and others may wish to take advantage of you, either sexually or in order to steal from you. If you allow someone you don't know that well to buy you a drink then attend the bar with them, or keep an eye on the transaction so that you can make sure you know what actually goes into your glass! Should you ever find yourself in the situation whereby you feel your drink may have been spiked, tell a friend immediately and drink water. Always keep an eye on your friend's glasses too and discourage them from accepting drinks from strangers. If you feel they have been spiked, don't leave them alone for a second. Call for help (a friend or family member who can collect you both) and inform the police or security. 'Date rape drugs' have a powerful anaesthetic effect, especially when they are mixed with alcohol and can take effect within minutes. They don't always have an unusual taste or smell, so if you start to feel strange, something may not be right. The effects of a date rape drug can last for several hours so it is important to get to a safe place as quickly as possible. Many people have someone who they can trust, be it a flatmate, friend, or family member. Call them, alert them of the situation and ask them to come to help you immediately, then call emergency services.

The symptoms depend on the substance used to spike your drink, but they usually include some of the following behaviours and reactions:

- Lowered inhibitions
- Difficulty concentrating or speaking
- Loss of balance and finding it hard to move
- Visual problems, particularly blurred vision
- Memory loss (amnesia) or 'blackouts'
- Feeling confused or disorientated, particularly after waking up if you've been asleep
- Paranoia
- Hallucinations
- Nausea and vomiting
- Unconsciousness

So no matter *how* you feel, in terms of shame or embarrassment, get help. Never leave a public place unless with the police or an ambulance crew. Or if you see your friend acting in this way call an ambulance, the police, and a trusted family member. Well-meaning strangers may offer to help, but do not trust them with transport or allow them to take the patient anywhere, even to the hospital, have an ambulance come to you right where you are. Never leave a friend who exhibits this behaviour, or leave them with a stranger. It is your duty to take care of your friends.

Designated drivers. It's a good idea to appoint a designated driver when you go out in a group. Should you see your designated driver drinking over the limit then *refuse* to get in the car with them and ask your friends not to do the same. Always make sure you have the number for a local taxi company to hand, or know the public transport routes well. Make sure too that you keep aside some money for the fare for all of your party. It's a good idea to keep a twenty pound or dollar note in a separate pocket or compartment of your purse, wallet or handbag that is used *only* in case of emergencies, this being one. Getting into a car with a drunk driver *is* an emergency situation. Imagine not only the consequences of getting into a life threatening situation, but also the shame or guilt of worse circumstances.

When you are a designated driver, honour your friends and don't even let one drop of alcohol pass your lips. It's better not to tempt yourself at all.

Keep a two drink maximum rule, keep to singles. We all know the damage caused to our bodies and how we endanger ourselves when we are over the limit and very drunk, but how about a complete loss of inhibitions and saying things we'll regret when we've had just one too many. While I know you might think it's fun to let your hair down and drink like a fish, there is a time and a place for that (if ever), and as a rule, you should **set yourself some rules!** Who wants to be known as the shy one who happily dances on tables once you are plied with vodka?

A person who wishes to remain in control keeps a two drink maximum rule. It's easier to know how much you've had when you allow only two drinks (when sipped slowly, two should be plenty). After two drinks is when our tongues often get loosened and we lose our poise. Be mindful of this rule, especially when on dates or at formal events. Public drinking is risky business for a variety of reasons, so respect yourself enough to know your limits.

Double the pleasure, add food. It's never a good idea to drink alcohol without first eating. The stomach is meant to handle the digestion of food and water, not alcohol. When you have food in your stomach it somewhat decreases and delays the effects of alcohol, helping your body to process it much slower and in turn means you won't get drunk on very little. Ply a drunk friend with water and carbohydrates in order to sober them up. Be responsible for yourself and eat before drinking any alcohol. Better yet, eat *while* drinking. Share some food. There is no greater pleasure in life than sharing good food and some wine with lovely company.

Mix it up with sparkling water or soft drinks. Make every other drink a soft drink. It will also help to keep your body hydrated. Some soft drinks can take their own negative toll on the body, laden with sugar and chemicals, so sparkling or still water is the better choice, but it is up to you. Just stay hydrated while drinking alcohol. It's an ironic statement but one that will save you from too much embarrassment and headache later.

Drink only the very best. "But I only get to have *two* drinks?" I hear you say, well, what if those two glasses of wine were the most utterly delicious glasses you've ever had? Would you rather down two bottles of 'cheap plonk', or savour two glasses of a *quality* wine from the best of the menu. With alcohol, when it gets pricey, you save yourself from things getting dicey. It shows great self-control to decide you are having only two drinks maximum, but you can spin that into a 'luxury' experience if you allow yourself some pleasure in the fact. You don't have to be a complete wine buff, or know a lot about the wine making process to order good quality tipple. A sommelier at your restaurant or a knowledgable waiter should be able to help you out, but go with what you like. Most people know if they prefer a Cabernet over a Malbec, there are plenty of resources available to research wines, grapes and provenances of vineyards and vintages. Learn to get a taste for the best. If you are going to enjoy it only a little, then at least make the experience meaningful. The same goes if you like beer, vodka or whiskeys. Just choose the best—or don't drink at all.

Look for culture, not the drinking culture. When we don't respect something we tend to abuse it, and alcohol is no different. People say they enjoy drinking wine or beer, but do you think they are still *really* enjoying it five pints or glasses in?

It is doubtful wine makers and sommeliers would be impressed to see their hard work and curated blends being used as 'liquid to inebriate'. No, they want you to *enjoy* it, to really appreciate the craftsmanship and the effort that went into creating something unique. Something to be enjoyed and paired with the perfect dish. There is no need to be a bore about it, but learning to take a step back from "that stuff that gets you drunk" makes one far more cultured. When you can experience not only the product, but the delicious cultural *activity* of savouring a nice wine or craft beer, consuming alcohol in this classier manner is worlds away from the sorry anti-social behaviour that crowds our pubs and clubs every weekend.

Don't know where to start? Swot up in the Sunday supplements. They almost always have a wine buff touting the best choices.

What to do when you have had one too many. We've all been there, feeling a bit squiffy. Our heads are spinning and our speech is running away with us. Unless you completely abstain from alcohol, it's likely it might happen to you again at some stage, so the point is this, **learn your limits**.

Before you accept an offer of a top-up or another drink, ask yourself; "Do I really need this, or can I sit this round out and have a soft drink or water?" This doesn't mean you are missing out, and the ship won't completely sail without you. For fear it might run out, we drink as much as we can, while we can. Perhaps this is just British culture, regardless, it's not healthy no matter your age or heritage. Think about getting some food too. Many drinking establishments offer food of some variety. Carbohydrates are your best bet, but if you find yourself in a pub with only a packet of crisps or pork scratchings on offer then ask a friend if they would like to go for some food. Plenty of party-goers stagger in and out of kebab and burger shops on their way home on a night out. Regardless of class, food is better than no food.

When you've really had too much and feel you are over the edge then **tell a friend**. If you suddenly disappear to the loo for too long and they know you aren't feeling right then chances are that they'll come looking to check on you. Plant the seed in their mind that things aren't one hundred percent with you and their care-taking instincts will/should kick in. Sometimes too, we just have to call it a night. Never decide to up and leave on your own, always tell someone you are going. Organise safe transport. Call an SOS to your parents, friends, family or neighbour to come and get you. In the worst case scenario and you really must make it home on your own, call someone who is sober and let them know you are going home, how you plan to get there, and to meet you if possible. Make sure someone knows where you are **at all times**.

Looking out for friends. You cannot be considered a lady or gentleman unless you put others first. This too extends to times where you may be drinking and having a really good time. No time on the dance floor, sexual attention, or having a 'good craic' is more valuable than your friend's safety. Sadly, when people get drunk they can make silly decisions. You have to look out for your friends, and under no uncertain terms should you allow your friend to:

• Leave with a stranger, no matter how much one insists they'll be okay.
• Have a one night stand. Not good.

- Drink until they vomit—this is just stupid.
- Exhibit ridiculous behaviour just because they're drunk. Sexy dancing, risqué picture taking, dancing on tables and flashing private parts all count.
- Flirt with a member of the opposite sex if they are taken. Help to remove the temptation if they seem to be struggling.
- Get behind the wheel of a car, or as a passenger with a drunk driver.
- Drunk dial or text—whether it's an ex or a boss, it never ends well.

If you try to help them avoid these things and the behaviour still goes ahead then you have to make it known to them when you are both sober that you are not happy about the situation. Say it with grace and speak from a place of love, stressing how worried you are and that your friend is putting themselves at risk.

If they persist, then you need to make a decision. Help them realise that this continued behaviour might be a mask for a deeper issue that they aren't dealing with. Or, decide that you can no longer keep their company. If every time you go out your friend's behaviour turns debaucherous, then question if it's really what you want to be associated with.

Surviving a hangover. Whether you've had one glass or four, there will likely come a day when you will suffer a hangover. Factors that might increase your chances are; the heat and humidity, your levels of hydration, whether you ate, mixing your drinks, what you consumed (some people react to certain types of alcohol), your age, and your current level of health.

In order to survive your hangover your body needs three things; rest, hydration and food. A hangover is a sign that your body can't handle what you gave it—it is poisoned, and so, you must do good by your body.

Here are some techniques for getting over a hangover. I know some people swear by fried bacon or a 'hair of the dog' (another drink? In my mind fighting fire with fire is a ridiculous concept). These tips below will not fail your body:

- Get fresh air, the body feels stale and oxygen is required to help our internal organs function properly, so open a window or sit out in the garden or on a balcony for a bit. If you can handle it, a gentle walk also does wonders. Wear sunglasses if it helps.
- Rehydrate, water is your best bet. You can't have too much, so just keep drinking! Orange juice or ginger ale is good too in small amounts.

- Sleep it off if you can, with a window open.
- Eat something, carbohydrates are best. If you really can't handle it then eat some dry bread slowly. Pick off pieces and challenge yourself to eat one at a time.
- Avoid drugs. It is tempting to battle a headache with paracetamol or ibuprofen but all you are doing is masking the pain—this being a signal that is alerting you to a problem, in this case severe dehydration.
- Vomit if you have to, but don't force it. Listen to your body, if it needs to expel what is poisoning it, allow it.
- Lastly, just deal with it! What's done is done. You may have to resign yourself to feeling pretty rough all day, but it's your own fault my friend. Just ask yourself, was it worth it? If it was and you have no regrets about your behaviour then give yourself a pat on the back and try not to drink as much next time. See how much fun you can have on one less drink.

In the words of some very wise people who have gone before us, "Less is always more".

Recognising a dependency on alcohol

People are great at denying they are alcoholics and of course most people aren't, but while they may not be classed 'alcoholics', a large amount of people are actually alcohol *dependent*. So how do you know if you are alcohol dependent, or how can you recognise someone who is? These are some signs that can help identify the problem.

Worrying about where your next drink is coming from. This of course is a very strong sign of alcohol dependency, if not alcoholism. If you find yourself worrying, or thinking about the next time you can get a drink (clock-watching) then that may suggest you have a dependency.

You drink every day, no matter how little. Your social life revolves around it. In Europe especially, our cultures and social lives do involve alcohol quite openly. People meet in bars, pubs or restaurants after work, or we like to head to the pub or to sporting events and grab a few cheeky drinks. If you find you are turning down invitations to places where drinking alcohol is unacceptable, or you find yourself strictly planning your leisure time to *include* drinking, then you may have a dependency. Those with alcohol dependency simply feel that doing anything *without* alcohol is 'boring' and may be quite vocal about it.

Not knowing when to stop. We've all been there, having too much. Part of the human journey is sometimes taking things a little far, 'letting go' and having a good time. Perhaps you've had 'one too many' on the odd occasion where you've done or said something you regret and caused a little embarrassment. However, if you find yourself in this state *every* time you have a drink then this is a warning sign.

Drowning your feelings. Do your feelings of anxiety, depression or suicidal feelings only dissipate when you drink? Heavy drinking effects the neurotransmitters in our brains that are needed for good mental health, and while drinking can help you to 'forget' your problem, you are only really covering up a problem with another one. This is how alcoholism can really get a hold of you and create an addiction. Mental health issues when mixed with heavy drinking are a grave concern in the health service because many young adults and middle aged people are using alcohol to self-medicate their anxieties and mental health issues instead of seeking the real help that they need.

Suffering from withdrawal symptoms. Experiencing withdrawal after drinking alcohol such as sweating, shaking and nausea which stop once you drink alcohol are a warning sign something isn't right. If you are worried you might be becoming dependent on alcohol then consider how easy you find it to go a few days or even a few weeks or more without drinking. Finding it pretty difficult to cut out alcohol mid-week or even going a whole weekend without extreme desire for a drink is a pretty clear sign you may have an issue. When it comes to anxiety, stress, boredom and depression, alcohol may feel like it gives you an instant 'boost' in the short term, but it will never really fix the underlying issue.

In order to fix these issues, you must first realise that they are there and seek help.

A few tips on personal safety

Violence is never something we should have to resort to, but sadly in this day and age many people roam this planet in a state of distress, anger, bitterness and miseducation whereby they think it is ok to take things by force or use violence to get what they want.

Many of us will witness some violence in our lifetime and sadly some of us on a daily basis.

Cultured ladies and gentlemen are not exactly the violent sort, but we *should* know how to handle and defend ourselves in situations that are life threatening. Self-defence classes are fantastic for boosting your self-confidence, raising your awareness of potential threats, and learning how to avoid conflict. If you find you really enjoy it then taking a regular martial arts class will help you even further. People who learn defence techniques are strictly advised that they must refrain from using them unless absolutely necessary as they are very dangerous, but you never know just when they are needed.

As for raising your voice, one should only *ever* shout to alert people of danger. When faced with any threatening situation, shout as loud as you can for as long as you can, a simple "Help me" is not sufficient. Shout about the situation you find yourself in. "There's a fire in the building, the flat is flooding, the lock is jammed, I'm drowning, my leg is trapped", etc. A course in personal safety and self-defence will teach you how to control your fear and anxiety in these situations in order to get help fast.

It's worth doing and will always be money well spent.

A true test for testosterone. Gentlemen, gone are the days of the duel, and it is no longer considered poor form to walk away from a challenge. Gents you especially may find yourselves on the receiving end of physical threats from obliging drunk males in pubs, bars and most likely at sporting events. While it is a good idea to know how to defend yourself, you should *always* choose to walk away. Civilised Englishmen are more than happy to do this. This is never meant to imply that you aren't a strong man capable of defending himself or his lady but nothing can better prove how smart you are and 'above it all' by walking away from that drunken monkey taunting you. As much as it may pain you to hear the jibes and jeers, the insults calling you weak and pathetic, by quietly walking away you are acting like a true gentleman! Doing so with a protective arm around the shoulders of any woman you are with is also highly attractive.

An intelligent man knows that fighting is undignified and the outcome is likely to be a night in the police station.

No gent would dignify loutish behaviour with a fight, or matching the disgusting insults thrown at him. Shake your head, collect your lady and your friends and move on. Your lady will not think you weak, but rather chivalrous if you sweep her off her feet and *out* of that situation. Standing there swearing and throwing punches just drops you down to the level of the boorish pub brawlers we English always frown upon—a stain on the face of beautiful Britain. Don't be that man. Have understanding and compassion for him and focus on keeping your woman, your dignity, and your physical body safe from these crude encounters.

Managing your temper

Ladies and gents, if you learn to master and manage your emotions then you will also be able to control your temper.

Everything you do, say or feel is managed by an internal bank of emotions. This bank is brimming with all sorts of joys and anxieties, hatred, love, judgements, and opinions. The true mark of a graceful person is one who can manage his emotions in all situations, no matter what the initial gut reaction may want to do.

Anyone who loses their temper, has lost control. You only need to look at two people fighting to see this, and you don't even have to look far, television shows and movies always have some level of fighting or conflict on every other channel these days. People love to observe conflict! We keep watching it so the TV companies keep commissioning and airing shows like these. What does that say about the harmony in the homes of the people who give it airtime? Homes should be considered a *sanctuary* from this negative behaviour, and moreover, why are we exposing our children to it? Is that what we are teaching children, that conflict is solved by fighting? Violence with words is the answer? Tempers teach people a lesson?

My mother-in-law's oft-used phrase is appropriate here; **"where there is conflict, someone feels threatened"**.

Remember that saying the next time someone shouts at you, or you are tempted to lose your cool. Who is the threatened party? The person shouting their head off, or the one keeping their cool no matter what bile and negativity is thrown at them?

It pays to be poised.

Life is a journey of learning to master yourself within your environment. When one accomplishes even the smallest of personal victories their life opens up to new possibilities, fantastic encounters and contentment beyond belief.

GALLANTRY & GRACE

Personal Potential

You are not defined by your situation, but by your potential

Good manners, gallantry, and grace are those seemingly 'little things' that people love about the English. When the characters in your life are demonstrating and upholding these virtues, things run smoothly, people feel valued, and life feels a little more pleasant. The English are known for their steadfastness, their reserve, quietness, niceties, self-control, and enduring faithfulness. These are beautiful qualities and really something quite wonderful in this new world of bright lights, with its unashamed and messy liberalism, fame-seeking, and fast living.

The English are also very 'poised', which is born from a dignified state of mind that is always stable and self-assured, well balanced, and consistent.

Considering more than a fair few of us suffer from a little social anxiety; when it comes to new experiences, poise is something everyone should try and cultivate. It gives you back control of yourself. A calm and collected control of one's self is very simply, the sense of inner peace and stability in the state of mind of someone with a sense of purpose, confidence, and intelligence to know how to handle themselves in *all* situations.

Quietness, gentleness, and refinement have long been tossed out with that baby in the bathwater. As such we have lost most of what we know about self-control and how to cultivate it.

Sound knowledge of poise and etiquette is the one thing we aren't born with, and is now coupled with a culture that values nor teaches it. We need to develop and learn it for *ourselves*, and while it may feel like an uphill battle, once you start climbing, the momentum feels rather wonderful. The Englishman has made his pursuit of self-improvement an art in itself.

To go about attaining poise, we do not put on airs and graces. Instead we look inwards to study our minds, our anxieties, our fears, our social misdeeds—and we purposefully *correct* them. Not explicitly for the benefit of those around us, but for ourselves first.

Wouldn't it be nice to walk into any room and know that you can handle (with grace) whatever is thrown at you? That you can be at ease, to know what to say to the right person at the right time and never put your foot in your mouth? Or to have the confidence to try anything in life without the fear of failure (because you know it isn't really a failure, just a lesson to be learned and identified as an opportunity for further improvement).

The right recipe for achieving poise

Poise isn't simply the act of sitting down one day and poring over an etiquette manual then reenacting the 'rules' like a robot. This is where hoping to raise ones personal standards only by surface value goes wrong, or becomes rather obvious and disingenuous. This empty practice of 'etiquette' is technically akin to darning holes in your knitwear again and again without seeking out the moths. A hastily absorbed 'self-improvement' method rarely works out in the long run, and so you must look at what is going on underneath to cause the issue, naivety or lack of confidence in the first place and let it envelop every fibre of your being.

When we spend so much time trying to impress other people by the putting on of airs and graces it all comes across as rather fraudulent. It's no use trying to promote something as refined when it's rather slapdash underneath and not aware of the beautiful quality and potential it has.

You must *care* about etiquette and gracious living. Not solely to use in order to get ahead or socialise with the right crowd, but to be the best version of yourself possible and achieve your true potential.

The following pages will take you through some of the most important constituents in developing poise, self-confidence, and good etiquette based on humility and assurance, not dazzling charm and correct fork placement.

The key to this whole exercise is to obtain a humble but positive belief in yourself and your good character. This is the marked difference between men and women, and ladies and gentlemen; the truly classy, and the nouveau pretenders. Those that follow the common ways of the world, and those that are set apart.

Enjoy the pretty accessories, flash watches, holidays and homes by all means, but be absolutely sure what's going on underneath is worth all that aesthetic Instagram-worthy effort. Appearances are one thing, but noble character, elegant poise, and humble gentility are something else altogether.

Poise means to have composure and dignity of manner, a balance of being, and tranquility of 'self'.

Now we've covered the nature of etiquette from the heart and mind, we will turn our attention to the outward appearance and what people will see when they look at you. Your air of elegance, poise and attitude towards the rules of etiquette will be clearly visible from how you simply hold your body and the movements it makes.

Rather an overwhelming thought, but the simplest of gestures can give the game away as to how you feel about people, the environment you are in, and how you feel about yourself.

Any good Englishman and Englishwoman knows that the *less* you say with your body, the better. We have perfected the art of steely, cool and calm body language and physical poise for good reason—the details of which and the reasoning behind them follow in these chapters.

Poise & Body Language

Correct poise

When you commit to learning to improve your mental state and raise your self-esteem, and have made the necessary changes on the inside, your outward presence must correctly match your new found personal attitude.

The way you hold yourself says a lot about your attitude, so whether making an entrance into a room, walking down the street, or waiting in a queue, the one thing that can help to give you a good head start is having impeccable posture and poise.

A person with great poise and posture appears comfortable in their own skin. Their demeanour and body language is open and warm, non-threatening and appealing to people of all ages and gender and in turn, this makes people feel comfortable in their presence.

The difference between posture and poise is that one is physical and the other mental. Posture is how you carry yourself physically and poise is how you carry yourself mentally, both are ingredients making up your *presence*.

Have you ever been around someone who carries themselves well physically, but you still felt a little uncomfortable in their company? Like they were repelling you in some way? This is because their posture and their poise don't marry. In order to be a true lady or gentleman, you must carry yourself well but also be engaging and warm so that people will want to be near you. You have to emit an energy that says, "I'm friendly and I am happy to get to know you" but at the same time it says, "I am confident enough not to be pushed around, I know how the world works. I am in control of myself both physically and mentally".

Let's take an example from both sides of the fence.

A confident person stands up straight and looks the world in the eye. Head is held up, back straight and there is an ease to them that makes *you* feel comfortable.

However, if they were to have a bit of a cocky or self-centred attitude, the nose would raise higher, or they'd have their head turned away from others. They would look down on you or through 'side-eyes', the nose not facing you dead-on when looking you in the face. Though their posture may be erect it will undoubtedly be 'shutting you out', with an unwarranted stiffness, or a limb crossing their body as if to draw a weapon. One shoulder would angle away from you to one side, thus creating a barrier between you.

Sometimes the media portrays or parodies a 'lord or lady' in this way. They promote a person of good-breeding as being one who thinks of themselves as better than everyone around them and very stand-offish. As if a wall or a barrier is around them protecting her from being 'spoiled' or dirtied in any way. This could not be further from the truth about what is 'proper' behaviour.

If you want to befriend people and come across as engaging, warm, and lovely, then there is no use in fussing and preening and 'sitting pretty' like a king or queen only to be seen to be doing so. To be considered worthy of people's attention and admiration for your affability, you have to *feel it* in your heart.

The posture and poise of a true lady or gent are always married. While you can have good posture without poise (it looks good on the outside, but inside is a crumbling mess), it won't make you a lady or gent unless you are determined to master your poise *as well as* your posture and vice versa.

As an adult you are always required to be 'on form' at some point in your day. This could be during the school run, the commute, in the office, or in your dealings with acquaintances. The point of making sure you are keeping it together and using poise to radiate your best self is not to hide any issues you may have, but to mask them where you may not *want* people to know about them. There is a marked difference in being human and being a big bumbling mess. Remember, we are learning to be English and polite here. Unless you are in dire circumstances, not everyone cares how you feel this morning, and you shouldn't really expect them to.

Timelessly English celebrities make a good study for evidence of how posture and poise marry. Current examples with fantastic posture *and* poise are Colin Firth, Kate Winslet, Liam Neeson, Emma Thompson, Rachel Weisz, Michael Caine, Helen Mirren, Emma Watson, Benedict Cumberbatch, Emily Blunt and Dame Judi Dench. They all carry themselves well and have an inner and outer 'collectiveness' that can only come with good grace and poise. They turn up to red carpet events to do a job, answer questions politely, smile and get on with it. They put their best self forward and perform a duty. Take your pick from the rest of 'celebrity' who, now you see it, aren't of that same class.

So, are you wearing your emotions, drama and thoughts on your sleeve? While waiting in a slow and long queue at the supermarket, you may be standing beautifully but does your face show what you are really thinking, are you huffing and throwing your gestures around to show your irritation? Slumping your posture out to one side, hand on hip and eyes rolling? Hopping from foot to foot in immature impatience?

It won't make the queue go any faster if you huff and puff and it only serves to irritate those around you. You lose your cool and lose your grace. What will the cashier think of you and how will he treat you when you finally approach the till? How do you *want* him to treat you and how *should* you act accordingly? If you want special treatment in life, you have to treat other people in the same way you hope to be treated yourself. They don't need to witness your drama, in your body language *or* your energy.

The same goes for friends as well as the public. At dinner with friends or family, or with a romantic interest, you may be sitting correctly and eating nicely, but if you are thinking about your financial concerns or about a disagreement you had with a friend, they will be able to tell. There is a time and a place to discuss these matters, and mulling them over in your head will mean you bring that energy to the meal with you. Unless you are in good company where you can discuss and perhaps try to sort these matters out, leave them at the door and enjoy the moment for what it is!

No one can make you happy but you, so never rely on others to do it for you —there's always a risk of disappointment. It is also common courtesy to not drag other people into your drama. So don't miss a beat, be gracefully poised at all times. Only when appropriate and in forgiving company can you let it all out! Pick your moments.

Have good posture dear

The benefits of correct posture are threefold. Our physiology performs better and as a result we ward off any future problems like muscular and skeletal aches. Many causes of joint pain and muscular spasms are down to poor posture, particularly ailments and misalignment of the back.

Where vanity is concerned, the best point of standing straight is that we also look good! The simplest way to look good is to look healthy and confident. We are attracted to lean, fit people with clear skin, white teeth and shiny hair —and most importantly, great posture. These are the indicators of health, both physical and mental. Correct posture also helps to give the illusion that you are slimmer than you really are. Hunching over only creates unsightly lumps, bumps and bulges where we really might not wish them to be.

Posture shows strength, an awareness of the body and inner confidence. Good posture makes you look supremely confident in your own skin which is a good marker for the state of the person's mental health.

When standing, it is good to think through all the points or 'marks' that you must hit in order to stand correctly. It may seem a lot to remember but if you consistently practice it will become second nature.

POSTURE, an acronym to remember:

P   peacock neck

O   open chest

S   shoulder blades together

T   tummy lifted

U   unbroken line in the hips

R   really straight, but soft knees

E   evenly distributed weight on the feet

To explain this acronym in more depth:

Peacock neck. In order to face the world and not the floor, our neck needs to support our weighty heads so that we can look straight on and actually see where we are going. People never really give the neck much thought but it is very important in your overall posture as it is the beginning of a nice straight stance. You are aiming for a nicely still, lean and upright position. Never completely stiffen your neck like a soldier at his post, but try to keep a straight neck with the underside your chin at a right angle to your neck, parallel to the floor. Holding your chin at a right angle to your neck also decreases the look of a double chin and avoids the 'nose in the air' look that people obtain when they are straining too much. Keep your neck vertical and your chin horizontal to the floor.

Open chest. Holding yourself with an open chest means that you will be less likely to hunch and you will be able to breathe better. Need I mention also the benefit to how the neckline of your clothing will improve. Women with an ample bosom often try to hide their size by holding their chest in a concave position and hunching the shoulders over but this only serves to give a heavier, not to mention droopier look, thus defeating the purpose of trying to hide the chest in the first place. Smaller busts too will be shown for the curves you do have rather than hidden and truncated. Necklines of dresses and blouses sit better on an open chest as they lie flat over the décolletage as opposed to gaping when one hunches. This helps to avoid embarrassing flashing incidents. Lifting the chest into an open position also visually separates the chest from the trunk giving the illusion of a slimmer waist and arms as they will be held further back on your frame. The 'roundness' is also reduced in the upper arms and at the top of the shoulders. For gentlemen, an open chest serves to make him look approachable, to lift the stomach area, and reduce any mid-section paunch.

Shoulder blades together. Moving the shoulders back and down works in harmony with the open chest. It keeps the spine in correct alignment and pulls you upright. With shoulder blades softly together, the head is held higher, the upper arms are held further back and you appear slimmer as a result. This also avoids strain in the shoulders (trapezius muscles) and neck.

Tummy lifted. When the chest is open and shoulder blades are together there is an increased sense of space in the stomach area. You naturally 'pull' the stomach up and in. Over time your muscle memory will begin to hold your waist in a trimmer way. Just as the stomach might have learned to be slack and paunch, it can also learn to hold itself in. Imagine ever so gently pulling the bellybutton in towards the spine rather than sucking it all up inside your chest cavity. Try some gentle Pilates exercises to really strengthen your core if you find this a challenge.

Unbroken line in the hips. So many women these days, I am guessing from taking cues from 'sexy' celebrities, or perhaps after having and carrying around small children like to stand with one hip 'popped out'. This is neither good for your posture alignment, your back and hip joints, or your look! It puts all your weight on one leg, often making it stiff and truncated, flattening the knee on the weight bearing leg and throws your entire balance off. When you are stood in correct posture there should be a smooth, unbroken line travelling up the leg, past the hip and into the trunk of the body. You shouldn't have any sharp angles or popped hips at all. This will take much pressure off your hip joints and help you to stand up tall as you should. I should mention also that it is easier to walk and 'get going' when you stand correctly as positions with a popped hip require that you first stand up straight before you can even propel yourself forward into motion.

Really straight, but soft knees. Standing erect like a soldier flattens your knees, making them look chunky and, it throws the weight of your body forward at the hip line. Both of your knees should be soft and pointing in the direction you are facing when you are standing still. Ladies, if you like to stand in a more feminine way as detailed further on, there are slight variations to the leading knee, but regardless of the way you stand, never throw your knee cap back into its socket as this can become rather painful and makes standing for long periods of time uncomfortable.

Evenly distributed weight on the feet. Make sure when standing, that you distribute your weight evenly over the foot. You should think of your foot like a tripod. There should be equal distribution on the heel, ball of the foot and foot pad immediately below the little toe. Of course, for ladies, heels will throw this balance off, however don't rely too much on the heel of the shoe or the ball of your foot to take your weight, try and aim as much as possible for the tripod. When wearing heels, if you are forced to throw all your weight on the ball of your foot with no possibility to distribute your weight back into the heel, then quite simply your heels are too high! There is also a very feminine way to stand that looks elegant and slims you down much more than standing straight on. If you like to stand straight on (considered to have more masculine energy and is a 'business professional' way to stand), then make sure you are placing your weight evenly over both feet so as to avoid the popped hip look and throw your line off balance. Keep your feet with toes pointing forward and neither too close together nor too far apart. About inline with the alignment of your hip bones is good. This option is detailed below to explain the posture further.

Standing for ladies

There is no denying that women from times past, and today's ballet, ballroom and latin dancers know how to move their bodies. Once taught by mother to daughter, and yes, in finishing schools, these tricks taught a woman how to do something as basic as standing, still hold a presence yet still remain feminine in their line, *and* draw positive attention from those around them. The fundamental standing posture is the same as explained previously, but the difference is in the placement of the feet and the distribution of your weight when you stand.

A feminine stance can make you look significantly slimmer as you are angled in such a way that it gives the illusion of a leaner silhouette—hence why models and beauty queens use it!

To start, stand facing a mirror with your feet together. Heels touching and toes pointed in the same direction. Make sure you correct your posture using the POSTURE pointers. Notice how you are standing nicely, but it is altogether rather 'square'. Men look great in this pose as it creates a sense of dominance and honesty (nothing to hide when you are facing the world) and for women in business this is an affective stance when you want to be taken seriously without question. For women interested in elegance, there is a nicer way to stand that will show off your feminine energy and make you appear leaner, more attractive and approachable. Above all, the main aim is to look serene. Busyness, fidgeting and jerky movements do little to help your cause if you want to look beautiful and draw attention.

Standing in an elegant way

A lady should stand in what ballerinas call third position. The look of a beginner ballerina is what we are aiming for, as too much turnout in the feet is extreme. This will mean your weight is still somewhat balanced on your back leg and your feet are at right angles to one another ('2' and '11' on the clock face). Your back foot at forty-five degrees from your body, the front foot's heel is in the centre of your back foot, about one to two inches away from it and also facing forty-five degrees in the other direction. There should be soft bend to the front knee. This creates a nice line through the hip on all women. Remember to balance on your foot's tripod for good weight distribution. The back foot should be taking about sixty percent of your weight, with forty percent on the front foot. The body line is still upright and relatively straight, and no obvious curve in the hip. A lady's stance is well balanced, yet soft.

Back foot. Your back foot bears a small majority of the weight, it is in a two o'clock position.

Front foot. Your front foot at the eleven o'clock position, with the heel of the front foot sitting against ball or centre of back foot.

Hips. The hips are mainly facing forwards with an ever so slight twist towards the leading foot.

Arms. Holding something (drinks, canapés or a handbag suspended by the elbow). Or positioned in front of you loosely clasping the hands. Never resting on a hip or with arms folded.

Standing for gentlemen

All gentlemen must aim to stand in a refined way which suggests good confidence without appearing too aggressive. One must always remain upright with chin parallel to the floor, with chest and shoulders square-on to the crowd or your conversation partner. The shoulder blades pulled together and stomach gently pulled inward towards the spine. Men in general have less concern with appearing 'wide' in the hip or thigh area and can stand with feet parallel to one another. Adopting such a straight-on pose exudes honesty and demonstrates engagement in the conversation. Any back-footed stance or twisting of the body from the hips or at the shoulders may indicate you are looking to leave. Gentlemen when standing must not, unless in a very casual or sporting event, put his hands in his pockets, fold his arms or rest his hands on his hips. If one is unsure of what to do with ones arms or hands, clasp your hands gently behind you in the small of your back as oft demonstrated by the Duke of Edinburgh. Be quick to release your arms to proffer a handshake at all times.

Sitting down

The average person sits for around eight hours per day. It's an awful lot of sitting and therefore important that you get it right for your health.

Have a think about the way the average person sits around on their sofas while watching television, they are usually quite relaxed. Lounging, feet up, slumped and curving the spine in all sorts of angles. Sitting with one leg tucked under you for hours on end. If you eat in this position, just imagine what this is doing to your poor digestive system.

This isn't to say you should never relax, but just take the time to think about whether your back and neck are properly supported and that you aren't cutting off circulation to parts of your body. If you sit with your legs crossed at the knee for example, you are seriously restricting the blood flow to the upper leg as the main arteries run behind the knee. In the long-run there is a chance you could develop painful varicose veins or deep vein thrombosis.

To sit gracefully on a chair of any sort, follow these easy steps:

- Approach the chair, stand facing away from it with your calves gently touching the edge of the seat. This is to confirm its distance and that you will indeed end up sitting on a chair rather than the floor. If someone is pushing your chair in for you from behind (usually a chivalrous date or waiter) then wait for the chair to make contact with the back of your legs before you start lowering your bottom.

- Remaining as upright as possible as you lower yourself, keeping your back straight, use your thigh muscles to ease yourself gently down. You shouldn't need to use your arms for this. Your thighs should do all the work to take you down and bring you up, with your back remaining straight, head looking forward. Try to avoid using the chair arms to heave yourself up or lower yourself down.

- Make sure you don't stick out your bottom or bend too much at the hip as you sit. For ladies, immediately after this lowering motion, your knees should move to one side as you sit, generally the left. Knees and ankles should remain close together at all points during this seating motion. Remember, no gaps between the legs! Ladies you may use your hands to smooth your skirt or dress under you as you sit if you are wearing one, but this of course isn't necessary if you are wearing trousers. Gentlemen undo your blazer or jacket button before you sit, and there is no need to sit with legs wide open once your bottom has made contact with the chair! Of course anatomy may dictate that you can't sit with legs crossed or completely together, but neither is it necessary to expose all and sundry to the undercarriage of your trousers. Sit with your legs as close together as is *comfortably* possible.

- Once seated, if you find yourself too far forward in your chair, you may slide yourself back ever so gently if you can manage it, or rise an inch or two to gently plop your bottom further back in the chair.

- Keep your weight as evenly distributed as you can over both sides of your bottom. If you are going to sit for a long time it's best that one side doesn't take too much strain and fall asleep. You can sit with your knees and ankles together facing forwards (though there is a risk here of some up-skirt peep shows if you aren't careful), or to the side (generally knees to the left) with the ankles together or neatly crossed.

- Never sit with your legs crossed at the knees. This is not a cardinal sin, but it is very bad for your health in that it causes vein and circulation problems. The possibility of varicose veins in later life isn't worth sitting this way. Aesthetically it also tends to squish the thighs together and adds 'bulk' where most women don't want it. I've often found it causes pins and needles after too long which isn't a great idea as twitching and jumping about to get rid of it, or limping to the bathroom because your leg is dead, isn't very graceful. Some feel that sitting with your legs crossed is very 'sexy', and while it may be so, it isn't very ladylike. You must make your choice about which camp you'd like to be (or sit) in.

Some gentlemen like to sit with one ankle rested upon the opposite knee. This is only acceptable in informal occasions and should never be a chosen way to sit when in a formal, public or work setting. Keep this relaxed seated posture for private homes only. Make sure to check for holes in ones socks!

In summary:

- Feel the chair with back of calves to confirm its distance.
- Lower your body with your back straight and thighs doing all the 'work'.

- Sit on the edge of chair first then slide back to the mid point.
- Knees and thighs should always remain together, like you are trying to grip a penny between them.
- Ankles together and in alignment with a leg of the chair. Cross ankles if you like, but never legs.
- Distribute weight evenly on your bottom for long term comfort.
- Hands should be placed gracefully in your lap or on the arms of the chair, never sat on or used to prop up your head.
- Don't put too much weight on the arms of the chair.

Walking

Good posture is essential to a great walk, and the correct alignment of the body can still be corrected even if you have been stomping about pigeon-toed all these years. Learning to walk gracefully is a good idea, not only for the positive image you will project but for your health too.

Not only is better posture and a healthy walk great for your body and mind but it will also make you look attractive! Great body language is observed when in motion too. Your walk is an indicator of self-esteem and elegance to all that see you pass by.

There are many types of walkers. The agitated and sprightly, the slow and stomping, the heavy and hunched, the stiff and uncomfortable, the 'sexy' look-at-me's, and the graceful. Graceful walkers are quietly unassuming but in no way a wallflower. There is no sense of bold sexiness to the walk, overall it is rather demure but very alluring because of a great sense of poise and inner confidence. Watch movies and footage of old Hollywood starlets and leading men (the graceful ones) to get a sense of the correct movement. Audrey Hepburn and Grace Kelly are great examples of relaxed femininity in their posture and walk. Most male actors who have been cast as James Bond are fine examples also. Modern examples are; The Duke and Duchess of Cambridge, as well as older generation classic actors such as Michael Caine, Helen Mirren and Emma Thompson. Study fine actors on how they walk and move when they are out of character and being themselves at award shows. No movements are jerky or awkward, with everything slow and graceful. Walking the red carpet and even raising an arm to wave to adoring fans is neither rushed nor awkward. The art of graceful movement is *slow* movement.

In order to walk and move correctly, you must first learn to stand correctly, which we covered previously—remember our POSTURE? First stand correctly, then using your leading foot (usually on the side of the body that you write with, left or right), propel your body into movement, making sure to keep everything else in your POSTURE engaged. Keep your head high, shoulders together and down, your back straight, tummy in, hips straight, and keep your weight evenly distributed over the feet.

Do not aim to strut like a supermodel or hard-man. You are looking to achieve a dignified and unassuming walk; nothing that brings too much sexual, aggressive, nor negative attention. Quiet confidence is the key.

The most important things to take notice of when walking are at specific points in your body and are outlined below:

Feet. Are your feet pointing forward? It seems like a trivial thing to concern yourself with but it really does set you up for a graceful walk if they are correctly aligned. Many people walk with either inwardly turned toes, or turned too outwardly. This not only looks awkward but can put incredible strain on your hips and lower back. It can throw you off balance and create a swinging or bouncy walk. Keep your toes pointing in the direction in which you wish to travel and above all make sure your weight is balanced on the tripod of the foot.

Heel to toe. The most efficient and healthy way to walk is heel-to-toe. This means that the heel strikes the floor first followed by a rolling movement through the foot towards the ball and toes. The last part to leave the floor is the underside of the toes. It is easier to walk in this manner when you are barefoot, or wearing flat or low-heeled shoes.

Wearing heels? While heel-to-toe is the most efficient and healthy way to walk, when a woman wears higher heels, this can significantly hinder natural movement and create problems both for the walk and the overall health of your body. High heels not only cause a shortening of the Achilles tendon and calf muscle over time, but walking incorrectly can also damage your lovely shoes!

Ladies, consider your heel height. High heels block the natural movement of the foot because of the depth of the pitch (the angle of the longest part of the shoe which sits directly below the arch of your foot). This unnatural angle is why you need to make some adjustments to your walk. Often, many women teeter about in heels, as if tip-toeing simply because their heels are too high. The steep pitch sends the weight of the body onto the ball of the foot and relies on the toe box of the shoe to do all of the work. When this happens, one cannot strike the floor with the heel first because it is in too high a position.

Quite often when a ladies' shoes are too high for her, she fears the stiletto heel will snap or they'll fall to the side and she overcompensates by throwing her weight forward to stabilise herself.

When trying on shoes in a store see if they fit the foot, but make sure to walk about to assess if one can sensibly walk in them. If you cannot roll your foot through a natural walking movement and trust the heel to take your weight then they are no good, and certainly not graceful. Pin-thin heels, too little support in the toe-box, and many unsupportive straps are the worst offenders, as is any heel over a three inch height. You need to be able to trust the heel to take your initial weight before you roll through to the balls of your feet.

However if you are so in love with a pair of shoes that you simply *have* to wear them then make sure you get a taxi directly to wherever you are going and that you sit close to the loo so that you don't have to walk through a crowded room and bring everyone's attention to your badly considered choice of footwear. People do notice when you can't walk in your shoes, and it isn't positive attention. Sorry to be so abrasive about 'high fashion footwear', but while it may be aesthetically pleasing, it is not attractive or pleasing for anyone to know that you made a foolish choice of footwear for the sake of vanity or trends.

This is not a graceful decision to make. Pretty practicality is far more becoming on a lady and her shoes tell you a lot about her sense of self-respect. Respect your feet and they'll respect you.

Alignment of the feet. It is not advised for a lady stand still with her feet hip width apart. This may be appropriate in an exercise class setting, but not for general day-to-day living. This stance is quite masculine and if one is a lady trying to appear graceful, ladies should avoid having gaps between their thighs at all costs. Standing with your feet hip width apart appears very square and walking in this manner gives you a 'ploddy' air. If there is too much of a gap between your feet when you walk your gait will be very heavy and masculine. The anatomy of a woman's body is set up in such a way that she should have a slight curvature and elegance to her walk. Don't fight it, women have shapely hips for a reason! Gentlemen, keep your foot alignment and gait straight with a natural smooth and certain movement in the leg or hip, you are not a tin soldier and shouldn't look as though cemented to the floor. Plodding and dragging of the feet is most unbecoming, keep footsteps light but sure.

One foot in front of the other. Ladies should aim to walk with one foot in front of the other, as if you are walking along an invisible line that both feet must touch when stepping down. This will give you a graceful walk and will feel most natural for the movement of a female body. Never overcompensate by crossing your legs in front of one another. This 'walk' is reserved for runway models only. Never a good look for a lady of elegance. Gentlemen should walk with feet close to this invisible line but the footsteps should not be placed immediately on top of one another. Imagine a painted yellow line in the road, walk with both feet making contact with the line on the inner side of the foot, but no step entirely on top of it.

Ladies, those hips won't lie. How you move your hips says a lot about you and can make or break an elegant appearance in seconds. Many know that the shape and movement of a woman's hips are linked to her sexuality and hips have been celebrated and emphasised in fashion and art for hundreds of years —a movement of the body which sets the sexes apart. Men have narrower hips, that face front and hardly sway when they walk. Women however have very curvaceous hips that sashay and swing and pop, rise and fall. Even those with very narrow hips tend to have this sense of swing in the hips despite the lack of curve. Ladies, by all means embrace this feminine movement but like all things, it is best kept subtle.

If you watch women beauty pageants, runway models or celebrities you will notice how they walk with a real swing to their hips and bottom. They are exaggerating the movement of the hips *because* they want to draw your attention to their femininity and sexuality. In the wrong setting this can seem inappropriate because value is only seen in what is shown—the body. A great tool for a woman who wants to rise to the top on merit of how sexy she is perhaps, but for a graceful lady who wishes to ensure respect then there should be no *exaggeration* in the movement of the hips. There is also no place for this type of body language in a corporate environment if a woman wishes to be taken seriously. We are quite simple creatures when it comes to subliminal messaging and attraction techniques. This overtly sexual physical display will distract male colleagues and threaten your female co-workers. Not a great way to make allies or gain respect in the workplace.

If you want to walk gracefully but avoid the 'come hither' signals, then it is your foot placement and stride that will control the sway of your hips, not the other way around. Keep check on your hip movement and consider whether you are swinging them for attention or because that is the way you naturally move. You'll immediately know the difference, as will others.

Stride. The ideal step length is about twelve inches from the toe of your back foot to the heel of your leading foot. This will achieve a nice, considered and even walk that is graceful and measured. Take your steps slowly and considerately. Why always in such a hurry? In today's society we seem to worship those who appear to be busy and in a rush all the time because busyness means success. Wrong! Success means that people wait *for* you. At work, I bet you walk alongside your boss at *his* pace. The same goes for the elegant of mind, if you control and set the pace, you control the situation. Try really hard to cultivate a sense of dignity and poise that shows you are in the moment and not just thinking about your next task, not desperate to keep up. It doesn't mean that you should be idle and slow, just considered and confident.

To illustrate the step distance, the heel of the foot you are walking onto should be roughly one foot's length in front of the toe that you are about to lift off the floor to step with next. The pace should be neither too fast or slow. A trick to consider your pace is to match it to the beat of a song. You'll need to practice this one, but take your steps in time with the children's nursery rhyme 'The Wheels on the Bus'. Every new word means a new step.

Arm swing. When running and moving fast, an energetic arm swing will propel the body forward in motion and adds additional speed, but if walking casually down the street or strolling around an art gallery then your arms need not swing.

Try to not move your arms more than six inches away from your body in front and behind when walking. You want a little movement so as not to appear stiff, but keep it graceful and polished. For ladies, holding a handbag to your left gives that hand something to do, and leaves the right free for shaking hands and opening doors. For Gentlemen, when walking alone keep hands free from pockets, and when with a lady proffer your left arm to the lady and keep your right free for holding open doors. Try not to make any sudden movements with the arms, taking care to move them artfully and in a dignified manner. You never know who you might accidentally hit.

Walking with a lady

Gentlemen, when walking with a lady, always offer your arm. If she refuses this is her prerogative, but if she accepts, offer the arm furthest away from the road so as to protect her from oncoming traffic. Should you need to remove her arm for any reason, do not simply drop it, but instead lightly grasp her hand with your free hand and lower it gently. Offering your arm again as soon as the opportunity arises. There is no age limit, up nor down, that dictates you cannot offer an arm. When walking with several women, offer first to the eldest lady. Take care when offering your arm to a married woman of similar age to yourself as she may find this uncomfortable. Be Gentlemanly and offer, but do not be offended if she declines. You should still make sure to protect her from immediate oncoming traffic by standing to the appropriate side.

Handbags and toting things

Most often we are carrying a *hand*bag when we are walking through a town doing *town* things. For casual days and errands cross-body bags are the best option as they use your body to cling your 'things' to you, leaving you able to move your body as you naturally should. They are also the least likely to be stolen. The practicality of a cross-body bag is the clear winner for almost all daily occasions, but we know that a lady likes her variety... Note that shoulder bags, totes and clutches require us to change our body movements and thus they may affect our movement.

When using a bag that is carried over the shoulder, try not to overcompensate the weight by leaning to one side. This is particularly bad for your spinal health and will make you look awkward in your movement. What exactly are you carrying around to make it so heavy? Clear it out!

Shoulder bags with shorter straps are fine as they sit under the arm at the side of the body, but try to avoid using bags that are too bulky or overfilling it so that it resembles a stuffed pillow. The frame of the bag should never be under any strain. This not only creates weight on your shoulder causing you to dip and 'hoik' the bag back on your shoulder all the time but it makes one arm stick out like a penguin wing.

Clutch bags are useful for the evening, but they should only carry pared down items. You should be able to comfortably carry and handle your clutch bag in one hand so the size and weight must not go against the concept of a 'clutch'. If you can't clutch it in one hand, it isn't performing the purpose. Paring down to a phone, keys, small wallet with cards and cash, and a lipstick should suffice. If you need or want to take anymore than that, then a larger handbag is needed. It's not a pretty sight to see a lady play and fail at a game of Tetris with the contents of her bag.

Totes, the absolute bane of the bag world. They are useful to tote everything one might need, and for this reason are beloved by all women, but unfortunately the things are jolly cumbersome and large. Understandably we all love them but need we carry them around on rigid arms held at ninety degree angles pointing out like weapons? Or due to the weight we carry them at the elbow with our fists clenched and held tightly against our chests for fear of the tote either slipping off our arm or someone snatching it from us? The major crime is the rise of the 'statement bag' that seems to require we carry it at such an angle so that it can be 'seen'. It becomes something glorified rather than simply a device in which to carry our belongings.

Women 'display' bags, ladies *carry* them. If you use a tote, consider emptying it once in a while so it isn't bulging, or too weighty. Alternate between carrying it down the side by the hand (they can hold things better than the elbow). If you must carry it at the elbow then don't make a show of it. Your bag is there to serve you, not the other way around. Look at how the Queen carries her Launer handbag. It is always there, but also gracefully held and inconspicuous. Ironically her handbag costs a fortune and yet she doesn't use it as a status symbol to display her importance and wealth. A lady should look at her handbag in the same way. Sure, they are items of beauty and there is nothing wrong with loving the design of a handbag, but don't let that be 'all there is' to you. When a handbag makes an entrance before her owner, not to mention leaving a better first impression, then the balance is off.

Walking on uneven surfaces

Every person has trouble walking on different types of surfaces and while it'll never be all that easy, or look elegant, there are some smart things that you can do to assist yourself.

Grass. Grass is everywhere. Mainly in gardens and parks where you will hopefully be dressed for the right situation in sandals, wellies or trainers. It is fashionable to hold weddings and parties in gardens when the weather is fair so it's likely you'll be tasked with walking and standing on it for long periods of time—ladies, probably in heels! If you have an idea that you will be standing on grass then be smart and choose the right footwear. Ladies may wish to wear heels to outdoor events, but make sure they are appropriate. Stilettos may aerate a lawn, but the mud just below that green, let alone the natural pigmentation of the grass will do the heel no favours whatsoever. Choose a wedge, or a chunkier stacked heel. You won't spend the time teetering about or clinging to friends because you are sinking. An option is to purchase heel guards (if the hostess hasn't provided these, of course). They are little clear plastic devices that slip over the end of the heel to protect you from sinking into the grass and give you more 'surface area'. While they aren't attractive in themselves, they make *you* more attractive for giving you your balance and dignity back.

Strappy heels and sandals which provide no support to the foot and threaten to slip off are also not appropriate for garden parties. Grass is uneven and that mixed with shoes held on by a string are a recipe for a twisted ankle.

If you find yourself in the unfortunate situation of wearing unsuitable heels on grass then there are some tricks that will help you remain upright.

Stand close to hard-standing. Lawns that meet paving, cobbles or gravel are likelier to be firmer at the edges (though this is not true of the edge of a flower bed). Venturing into the middle of a lawn is a dangerous feat, the water often pools in the middle when it rains and so the ground will be softer making you much likelier to sink. If the grass is particularly long then it also indicates that the weather has been very wet recently. If it is shorn and dry then you have a good chance of it being firm. Like in horse racing, learn to identify what 'the going' is.

Balance your weight towards the front of your foot—it isn't good for you, but it might stop you falling back into the grass. Obviously make sure this leaning forward doesn't make you expose too much up top—gaping necklines are at the mercy of your posture, and if all else fails, admit defeat and take your heels off. In very polite company or at formal parties this will be frowned upon, but you should have thought about that before you chose fashion over form. In casual settings go for it and make a joke of it. Just don't traipse in and out of someone's home and trample mud into their carpet, and of course, watch out for hazards on the ground like glass, mud and gravel that are never kind on the feet. Think garden party, think flats or wedges.

Gentlemen: As it's likely you will be wearing sensible flat shoes, offer your arm to any lady you see in peril for support as she stands or walks across uneven terrain.

Cobblestones. Often found in market towns, places of interest and churchyards. Likely you are visiting for culture, in which case appropriate footwear is required. If met with unexpected cobblestones and you are in heels, then it's tiptoes and measured slow steps to the rescue! Need I say that if you pass by cobblestones every day on the way to work or school then take extra footwear. Precarious balancing is consistently risky, and also not kind to your shoes.

Slippery floors. A risk for all—there is not much you can do aside from praying that you won't fall. Go slowly and carefully even if you are in a rush. There's no point in breaking your neck over it. For some reason, many manufacturers (mainly those using cheap production methods) like to make shoes without any sort of grip. Always assess this when shopping for shoes, and if you find yourself in love with a pair without a suitable sole, then for goodness sake, do something about it before you wear them! Score the soles with a pair of sharp scissors, a box grater or rough sandpaper. Or you can take them to a cobblers and ask them to glue thin rubber soles on (the best option for safety). Or, as I like to do, slip them on and find your nearest patch of rough ground like gravel or a paved driveway, then stand there and keep dancing 'the twist' until you feel you've worn down the sole and the heel enough to provide you with a safe step.

Ice and snow. Invest in a good pair of walking boots. Wellies, while good for wet weather are no good in the snow as the grip on the soles are no match for compacted ice. You can also buy 'ice grips' that will slip onto any shoe to provide extra assurance. Make sure you purchase these from a good outdoor/leisure shop and take in the shoes you intend to add them to. Loose or ill-fitting grips are just as dangerous as no grips.

There is nothing more frightening than watching people trying to commute or make errands in icy weather wearing heels, office shoes or trainers. Though you might live in a country where snow and ice are infrequent, it never hurts to have a good pair of shoes meant for inclement weather. Adults: your feet have mostly finished growing by the age of fourteen so there is no excuse not to invest in a good pair of boots for bad weather that you can keep for a lifetime provided you take good care of them.

Getting in and out of cars

Getting in a car should be tackled backwardly, as in, your bottom gets in first. With the door open, turn to face away from the car, or at a slight angle facing away from it, and using your hands to steady yourself on the frame of the roof or door gently lower yourself in, bottom first, head ducked to avoid banging it. Once your bottom is on the seat, keeping your knees together swing them up and in.

Getting out should simply be exercised in reverse. Open the door, turn your body towards the direction of 'out', feet together swing them out of the car and place them on the floor, then using the seat or frame of the car, use your feet and legs to lift you up and out. Obviously you will have to bend forward slightly so that you avoid banging your head on the roof of the car (ladies; try not to bend more than needed if you are wearing a daring neckline).

In the waiting line

Waiting can be frustrating of course, but it needn't ruffle your feathers. Having the right mental attitude in these situations can help you keep your cool and your charm.

Quite often these situations tend to make us tired and irritable but that should be no reason for you to let it look so, for when you feel irritated, bored and annoyed it shows in your body language and you can look quite petulant. How many people have you seen waiting around in queues who look downtrodden and bitter? With sour, vacant expressions, eyes downcast at the floor, or worse, eyes rolling, they lean against walls, perch on dirty surfaces and begin to pick at their nails. The worst offenders are those who think that since they have a bit of time to spare, they decide to 'camp out' and spread their entire body and belongings all over the place.

When you queue, stand in your own personal space, not too close to the person in front (sadly, you cannot choose how close the person behind you stands). Make sure your body is pointing towards the area of focus, for example a service desk or counter. Turning your back on it or not paying attention will annoy others as it gives the impression that you are slow to react. Facing forward means you are always available for eye contact with the person serving. In some instances you may be seen first, or given information about wait times, etc. It leaves the opportunity open for communication. Don't flail your limbs all over the place and certainly don't huff. If you must 'do something' while waiting, then reach for a book rather than a phone and do look up from it from time to time. If the queue is short and doesn't require you to pass the time, then definitely do not take out your phone and scroll through it 'just because', you are better than that. Pay attention to those serving, those around you and your body language.

Arm placement

When feeling nervous, "What do I do with my arms and hands?" is a common thought. If you allow this concern to consume you, you'll wear this emotion in your body and people will be able to *tell* that you feel awkward and unsure of how to hold yourself.

If you are at a social function, then it is likely you will have a drink or canapés in your hand. Make sure to hold any items in your left hand allowing your right to remain free for handshakes. When your right hand is redundant you can either gently clasp your other hand (with the drink in it) or let it hang to your side. Ladies, if you have nothing in your hands gently clasp your hands together in front of you. Clutch bags oft save the day to allow your hands something to 'do'. Make sure to not cross your arms, or hold them behind your back. Both have negative body language connotations. You will look stand-offish or untrustworthy. Gentlemen, your options are a little limited leaving them to be clasped in front or hanging by your side if you do not have anything to hold. Regardless of your gender, best you make yourself busy or throw yourselves into conversation, it will soon take your mind off the trivialities of what your hands should be doing.

Posing for photographs

We all have a certain level of vanity and wish to portray a permanent record of our youth. Have you ever seen photographs of your parents and grandparents in their youth? What do you notice? They weren't exactly taking selfies with duck pouts, or making bunny ears behind the heads of their friends. No, they were photos taken of moments of time *that mattered*. Family or solo portraits in lovely settings and even the candid shots looked relaxed yet elegant. In our selfie-obsessed society we have forgotten how to have portraits taken of us. We so often rely on the reverse camera so we can pose until we get it right. Grandma didn't have that luxury, her photos were often taken with one or two frames, and yet she still looked beautiful. So how did she do it?

For a flattering posture. Standing with your feet together, take one step back on your dominant foot. If you are right handed, this may be your right foot—whichever foot you generally use to lead your steps when you walk. Your dominant foot and leg is stronger, which is why you are going to use it to support your weight.

Now, angle that foot at a forty-five degree angle away from yourself. So if you are on your right foot, angle it at forty-five degrees towards the right. You want to keep all of your weight on this back foot and leg. If it were a clock hand, your toes would be pointing at '2'.

Ladies: Taking your other foot, place the heel of that foot against the ball of your dominant foot. Your toes should be facing at '11', on the clock face. There should be no weight whatsoever on the passive foot (the one in front). Twist the passive foot slightly so that the inside of your foot and heel is facing slightly forward and your passive knee is crossed in front of your dominant leg. Making sure that your thighs are crossed. There should be no gaps or light visible between your legs. The passive foot should bear no weight whatsoever. You will notice that your hips are now angled ever so slightly to the right (or left, dependent on your dominant foot). Make sure you keep your tummy lifted, your chest open, shoulder blades together, shoulders down and your neck long. You can point your toes on the passive foot if you wish, as though you were showing off the top line of your foot. This looks pretty. But is perhaps a bit too much of a glamorous pose for every day. It will however come in useful when you are ever on stage or anytime you are being photographed in a formal sense.

Grooming. Is your hair nicely kept and are there any glaring slips of make up? Sort it out if so. Don't make it a major grooming session but a quick straighten out won't be frowned upon. Aside from that, are your bra straps showing, is your tie or skirt straight, and are you all tucked in? Is any skin exposed that you don't want to be? Is your body language elegant and confident? Standing or sitting slightly at an angle to the camera, rather than straight-on is flattering for most. Concerning the face, the smile and the eyes are most important. It's hard to hold a smile for long without it looking forced so a good trick which almost guarantees a genuine smile is to shut your mouth and stop talking. Photos taking mid-chat are rarely flattering. Get your body and head into a comfortable position, then relax and close your eyes. Wait for your photographer to say "Cheese" (or whatever warning they may give), then quickly open your eyes, focus on the photographer, sharply inhale through the nose (which lifts up your posture) and smile—baring teeth, or not, is up to you. Doing this gives a warm 'new' smile and photographs your eyes beautifully. Seeing as you've just had your eyes closed, it's less likely you'll blink when the shutter goes.

Practice in the mirror and don't be afraid to use this technique when having portraits done. It's not a bad thing to want to look your best on permanent record.

Informal photographs are pleasant to look at and fun, but do bear in mind 'what' you are doing when they are taken. Friendly group photos of you hugging your pals are lovely, but pictures of you all pretending to hump a lamppost after a few too many glasses of wine might be funny at the time, but do you want those images turning up for the rest of your life? The same goes for stupid faces, some turn out okay, others are downright horrific—you need to make your choice. Just don't be that person who chooses never to smile in photos because you think it makes you look better, it doesn't. It makes you look miserable and you'll end up with an album that your grandchildren will look back on and wonder why you were so sour all the time. Photographs should be joyful and used to capture beautiful, tender and loving moments, not to document your vanity.

When you really hate a photograph taken by someone else then politely request they delete the photo, or try for another. If they insist you look fine and the contents of the photograph aren't damaging to your character then you may have to admit defeat, but if someone is holding you to ransom over a photo of your 'sexy dancing' on a table with your pants on show then there are two lessons here. Make better friends who respect you enough not to photograph you in those moments, and need I say it, don't get caught doing it again! Especially as cameras are *everywhere* these days.

There is no shame in having portraits taken professionally for you to use online if you want to be viewed in the best light. Celebrities have encouraged our vapid '1,000 pictures of me' culture encouraging many ordinary people to display hundreds of selfies on social media. The elegant of mind are wary of such obvious vanity and refrain from the pressure to join in. Just because you can, doesn't mean you should. In years gone by, polite society would have a portrait of themselves commissioned at certain key moments in their life, in oil or in photograph. This would have been a coming of age portrait, perhaps a wedding portrait, or one with their small children. There is nothing to stop you from commissioning the same from a photographer. Quite often they have hair stylists and make up artists on hand to help you look your best and the photos can be used as gifts for your adoring grandparents. To keep them timeless, keep them slightly formal. There is nothing stopping you from using them on social media and as professional online profile pictures (but not all throughout your feed). You need not be the lady or gentleman who updates their profile photo every week. A well taken portrait over one hundred ill-taken selfies speaks volumes about refinement and values.

Marital status and body language

Have you ever noticed that body language is talked about while dating or finding a partner, but not when one is spoken for? We'll only touch upon this vast subject briefly, but this minefield bears thinking about, whether you are interested in finding a date or are already taken.

The most important time to recognise your body language is when you are in a committed dating relationship, engaged or married. It shows great respect to your partner and yourself to not unwittingly encourage attention or romantic approach from other people.

Aside from wearing a sparkling rock or gold band on your left hand, there is not much you can do as a material token to demonstrate your relationship status apart from your body language. When a woman is available for approach she will often 'make eyes' at men, dipping her chin slightly to look through and flutter her lashes. She will sit in a provocative manner with her legs crossed at the knee in order to accentuate her curves and play cat and mouse with her eyes for attention. Looking at him, then looking away, only to return her gaze again. Men will often play the same gaze-look away game with a woman he is interested in. If the stolen glances are reciprocated then by all means approach.

If you are out with your date, you shouldn't be making prolonged eye contact with anyone else. Your body should also be facing them as much as possible.

Leaning in and gentle touching shows others that you are there only with them. If you are taken but out on your own or with friends, do not 'amp up' the sex appeal or catch eyes with the opposite sex. If someone should be appearing to try and catch your eye, of course give them a friendly quick smile (no need to be rude) then flick your attention elsewhere. Look at someone else in the room or at some*thing* if you are on your own. Give them no further reason to approach you. Your body language shouldn't be 'sexy' or trying to be, and if you get up and go to the bar or to the loo then don't make a scene of it, pay attention to the task at hand. If anyone approaches you to flirt or ask you out, be polite but firm with an unquestionable response such as: "Sorry, I'm married", or "I'm very flattered of course, but I'm taken". Be kind in your reply *without* a playful tone to your voice. No need to explain further. They'll soon get the hint, and if your date is with you they'll be pleased you were polite yet showed disinterest, and respected their status as your beau. Should they persist, remove yourself from the presence of the pest.

Gentlemen, if you are looking for a traditional relationship then *you* are the one to approach a lady and to do the chasing. Look for and be aware of the signals detailed above, but be mindful of staring *too* much. There is a difference between a smouldering look and staring, leering, elbowing and whispering to your mates. Wolf whistling or commenting on the beauty or body of a woman passing by is *never* acceptable. These boorish actions are off-putting to a woman—it smacks of immaturity and is completely tasteless.

Regardless of your company or hers, always approach a lady alone. You don't need a wing-man. If your intended lady is with a group of friends, approach and talk to her directly but do not separate her from her group. She will separate herself if she is interested, but do not suggest it yourself, and never take her too far from the group she arrived with—a table over or a few feet away is fine. Give her a way out and a way back if she needs it! If she is drunk, by all means get chatting to her on a friendly level but do not ask her out immediately. You want to assess her behaviour and self-control before diving in, not to mention avoid any drunken situation that might get you both into trouble. Strictly no kissing or touching but do flirt with your conversation to show her you are interested. The invitation to go on a date can and should wait until both parties are sober. If you are both clear-headed and she refuses your offer of a drink, a date, or to give you her telephone number do not take offence, and absolutely never insult her verbally because of it.

Never take a refusal to heart, there is someone for everyone and not every woman will fancy you. A dent to your confidence it may be, but a polite and cheerful way of dealing with rebuff is sexy and intriguing. Don't question her decision, and make sure to pay her a genuine and nice compliment that leaves you both feeling good about yourself before you depart, such as; "Well, he's a very lucky man whoever gets to take you out". Then smile, turn and walk away. It is incredibly respectful, and you never know, it may intrigue her and she'll change her mind.

Taken ladies and gents, sometimes you may be out and about with single friends who are looking to date and you may soon find yourself in the company of the opposite sex (hopefully only briefly, as it would be rude on your friend's part to switch their attention towards a potential date for the entire evening). If one of the other party starts to flirt with you then drop tidbits about your single friend into the conversation, turn the attention off you and towards a single friend. Of course, bring up your boyfriend/ girlfriend/spouse in the conversation too, but don't bang on about them, they'll get the hint. There is a fine line between declaring your relationship status and being a bore to a wingman or woman. They may be there just to keep you company while their friend chats up yours, so keep it polite and friendly but anything but flirty.

"I'm available" body language is a tough one to get right as *obvious* flirting body language so often looks just that; obvious and anything but graceful! A lady worth her salt will not rely solely on her body to catch the attentions of a man because this is too carnal a way of finding a suitable date. Think about what you really *want* in a man, do you want him to treat you like a sexual object, or a lady?

Weapons of choice for the lady are her eyes and her smile, her charm, personality, intelligence, humility and grace. Not the legs, breasts, or bum. Live not by the patterns of the world and the hordes of man-hungry women around you who strut about bars in order to catch the attentions of just any man. You want the *right* man, and he won't be won with sex signals.

Gentlemen, avoid the ladies hamming up the sexiness, and instead approach the woman you find beautiful and charming. Not the easy girl who might give you what you want tonight. Are you looking for a woman for now, or a lady forever?

'Common' ways of meeting a girlfriend or boyfriend has had its time in the sun, and *easy-street* leaves little time for romance. Do everything in your power to choose an elegant love affair worth remembering, not a messy sob story.

Whatever you do, look up!

Keep your head high. Studies have shown that those who look 'up' when they are going about their daily lives are happier people overall. Look up! The best things are up there in the bright blue sky, they are ahead of you, outside of you, all around you. Only the saddest things are under you. Look ahead and look up, always.

Good Health & Gastronomy

To dine is to refine

This is where our lesson gets really tough, and we take absolutely no prisoners but as you read this chapter you'll realise it's for your own good. If you take note of the suggestions here listed you will not only level up in self-mastery but you'll gain an enriched lifestyle. It's time to pull your socks up and take some responsibility for yourself and your health.

For too long there has been much talk about positive body image and feeling good in your skin no matter what size you are. It is wholeheartedly agreed that we should learn to love ourselves, but this message sometimes muddies the waters as an excuse to abuse your body. It is a grave truth that the larger your waistband the greater your risk of onset diabetes, heart disease, cancer, and other weight related issues. Not to mention a long holiday to an early grave. So many of our modern diseases can be significantly reduced, if not eradicated if we simply took responsibility for the *quality* of our diet.

Too many children (those young and adult) have been left without parents because of a lack of care and self-discipline when it comes to personal health. Not to mention the children subjected to greater risk of long-term health problems because of an unbalanced diet at home.

This is not to say that we shouldn't enjoy our food, a good glass of wine, chocolate, or cheese board but we *must* learn to measure our gluttony for the sake of ourselves and our children. We must discipline ourselves in the art of self-control in order to release the grip that your appetite has over you.

The way in which you care for your body, not just what you clothe it in, or slap on it, is the *visual evidence* of how much care you have over your wellness, your level of self-discipline and importantly, when it comes to your children, how much you truly care about them. Sweeties and chocolates on demand, or for bribery, does not equate to love. It shows a lack of control, an inability to nurture, and poor demonstration of self-love and health education.

Take a look at the monarchy as an example, who by now you realise are our unofficial head boys and head girls of British society. We rarely, if ever, see ill health and obesity among them. The same rule applies to their children. Sporting pursuits and an outdoor lifestyle including riding and walking are encouraged to remain fit (not hours stomping away on a treadmill). Where we might imagine the royals eating caviar for breakfast and the richest of puddings at every turn, it is well documented that the Queen, and especially Prince Charles, are very modest and healthy in what they choose to eat, they prefer organic where possible—English grown and sourced of course.

So there we see trim healthy bodies, capable of withstanding long hours and stamina to rival a racehorse. The royals eat in a very old-generation way. After the second world war food was still scarce with rations remaining in place for a few years after peace was made. Indulgences were few and far between, portions were modest and food was local and seasonal. In stark contrast, this modern world with its 'have it all now' lifestyle is rapidly destroying our health. A mindset of modesty in all things is a good place to begin changing your attitude towards food.

The royals and any English families of 'good means' may have cooks, but the food isn't extravagant by any degree and could be accomplished quite easily by even the most average home cook. Note also the standard fare offered at any English boarding school and you will see favourites of the English palate which, in its most basic form almost always boils down to 'meat and two veg, plus a pudding'. It is also commonly referred to as 'nursery food'. An Englishman could quite happily survive on a diet of porridge & fruit, eggs & toast, or cereal with a good cup of tea for breakfast. A sandwich of choice with fruit and perhaps a yogurt for lunch. Any further snack may be fruit. All followed by a good home cooked meal of meat and two veg (in any guise), finished off with a nice stodgy pudding. A slice of cake or a biscuit on the odd afternoon and wine with dinner at the weekends make for a jolly nice treat.

This is all we really need to sustain our largely sedentary modern lifestyles. Exercise therefore need be little more than a thirty minute brisk walk thrice a week. Only greed (or a demanding physical job) will suggest you need more food than this of a day, and vanity the need to sweat it all out in a gymnasium.

If you wish to eat more, then your exercise levels must match the additional intake. It is as simple as that.

There is very little excuse for being excessively overweight. Science has proven time and time again that obesity and disease are triggered by personal environment and personal *choice*. The genetic disposition or preference for obesity and disease may lay dormant in your genes, but your lifestyle *choices* are the switch that activates them.

Before the witch hunt starts, this is not fat-shaming, this is health-giving advice and a much needed stern wake up call coming from a place of love. Sometimes one must be stern and 'cold light of day' honest—though not cruel —in order to be kind. Saying things are okay, or glossing over tough to address subjects for fear of offending isn't helping our first world nations to improve upon the population's health and unburden the health system, is it?

It is not shameful to be overweight, but it is an overwhelming shame to not do anything about improving your health and merely hoping medicines and quick-fix solutions will remedy any weight related health issues. We have one life to live and we owe it to ourselves and our children to make it a good one. That includes being able to enjoy *all* that life offers, not having to sit it out because we can't keep up.

You frankly have the choice to be healthy, you simply need to put down that chemical laden and sugar filled processed food!

Gourmet or gourmand?

Like bread and butter, self-control and a good diet go hand in hand. The fact of the matter is, unless one really has some level of will and self-control over what is put in the mouth, then a 'diet' to lose weight will never stick. For this reason we all need to learn how to make better *lifestyle choices* if we wish to enjoy good health. By proxy, this decision will gift you, as if by magic, a healthy and trimmer body in return. You needn't be as lithe as a supermodel or as ripped as a body builder in order to be considered healthy, in fact, a little meat on the bones is good for a person—but too much is most definitely not. It's about finding the right balance, and using good self-etiquette, and being kind to yourself.

You may wonder why this topic should be included in an etiquette book, or what it has to do with the English lifestyle, but remember that many of your **social** experiences *will* involve food of some sort. Your daily life certainly involves interaction with food. If you wish to have a refined life, then as well as your manners, your relationship with food is something you must also consider, critique, navigate, and master. How you treat the stuff you stuff yourself with, or rather, how you let it treat *you*, says a lot about your character, self-control, and willingness to expect and uphold the best standards in life.

One way in which to gain control over a gourmet lifestyle is to raise your standards in every area when it comes to food. There are a few simple choices that will help you to have a better relationship with food, better health in the long run, and an enjoyable experience every time you eat.

This is not rocket science. The following tried and tested methods have been hashed out in lifestyle books over and over again but the very crux of the matter is, *they work*. They are not diet tips, they are lifestyle choices.

The first two rules are simple and ongoing:

Eat only when you are hungry. This is the harder step to master as many of us rely on food for comfort or to relieve boredom. Try replacing misguided eating habits with a hobby. Getting lost in a good book, meditating, or time in prayer, taking a walk in nature or around town are positive ways to work through whatever caused you to reach for the biscuits. Make sure your habit replacement *nourishes* the body or the soul. It doesn't have to be taxing, just simply something to take your mind off food and give you space to think about what is making you feel you want to eat outside of meal times, or to comfort your feelings, and how to address it pragmatically.

Avoid junk and chemicals. Fast food is convenient for time but wholeheartedly inconvenient for your *body*. It would be impossible to expect anyone to cut out fast food completely. However you should do everything in your power to ensure that at least 90% of your diet (your three meals a day, plus snacks) are made up of fresh, whole, and home cooked foods. Save takeaways and convenience meals for when you really need them, or perhaps to enjoy on a celebratory occasion. Ordering a Chinese takeaway once a month, or on a birthday will do no harm, but indulging weekly is not a healthy habit. If you struggle for meal ideas or don't know how to cook, search for guidance on the internet and find out! Pinterest and YouTube are great resources for the budding cook. Why not indulge yourself and expand your horizons by taking a culinary course? If finding time is your issue then set aside one day per month and batch cook, portion up, and fill your freezer. Freezer meals that are home cooked with ingredients you can pronounce are far better than devouring an overpriced freezer meal that will also flood your body with high levels of salt and sugars.

The third rule is a wonderful adventure:

Raise the standards of *everything* you eat. Choose only the very best. Regardless of budget this is a choice that will ensure you eat very well, but in the right amount. Your budget may restrict you here and there, but when you learn to truly *taste* food rather than to simply consume it, the pleasure is increased, you savour it slowly, and therefore you will not require as much. Do you remember the last time you had a seemingly small, but truly indulgent pudding you couldn't finish because it was so rich? That is the experience you are looking for with the produce you buy.

Learn about food preparation and cooking methods by watching cooking shows. Read the supplements in the Sunday papers to get inspiration about what is in season, and find information about new products and tastes or dishes to try. Get to know your local producers, butchers, bakers and vegetable growers and let them *teach* you about their produce. Place priority on buying from local artisan food producers who pour love and passion into their production, rather than diverting your grocery budget towards conglomerates who care more for profits to line their pockets than public health and food quality.

Yes, this may mean a slightly more expensive wedge of cheese over the mass produced supermarket own-bland, sorry brand. Yes, this may mean three squares of luxury chocolate over three sugar-filled bars from a selection box. Yes, this may mean one beer over a six-pack. Or 'just' sharing one delectable, highly recommended bottle of wine instead of two cheap bottles of bottom-shelf plonk.

You owe it to yourself to live your very best life. If that means indulging in and *having* the best—but in moderation—then isn't that a more enriching experience than having a life full to the brim of things with zero value? In the words of Vivienne Westwood (who applied this phrase to fashion, but it works well for all things), "Buy less, choose well". *Fall in love* with food, and be passionate about it, but like all things that surround you, treat it with the dignity, respect and honour it deserves. Food is a blessing and not something to blindly ignore as you pour it down your gullet. Learn to savour the best of *all* things in life.

Lastly, learn to eat well. A finishing touch for improving your gourmet experiences is to use the good china! Set a nice table, drink from the crystal, put on a little music and eat by candlelight. If you don't own a full set of fancy china, it doesn't matter! Pieces can be picked up individually and at reasonable prices in sales, and even secondhand. Just because you might live alone or are starting out does not mean you should miss out on quality experiences. Buy one beautiful porcelain plate, one gorgeous crystal wine glass and a set of silver plated cutlery just for you and grow from there!

Remember to always eat at the table and dress for dinner! You needn't turn up in an evening gown and dickie-bow, but do make a little effort. Everyone enjoys eating together and the conversations and kinship that arise from doing so. Therefore pull your socks up and use that table for the reason it was created. A family that eats together sticks together.

Take time to relax the rules every now and again for good balance. A pizza party on the sofa with your lap as a table does no harm on occasion. Just take care not to slip into a routine of laziness as it takes the focus off what is on the plate and you'll end up losing sight of the very blessing that you have food to eat.

Table mindset and manners

Eating should always be a pleasurable experience and something to enjoy communally. In light of our lesson regarding improving health, no one really wants to hear about your boring diet at a dinner party. You are all there to be sociable and have a good time, not talk about the things you "can't have" or how certain foods affect you or make you feel.

Should you find yourself on a healthy eating plan and then faced with the minefield of a dinner party or social event surrounding food, your positive attitude and the lack of detail you impart on the matter is the most important way to exercise good manners.

Your host or hostess should have inquired about any dietary requirements before the dinner party, and if so, leave your trust in their hands. Finding yourself at an impromptu gathering is a little more challenging. If you have a food allergy or intolerance you can let this be known quietly to whomever is cooking or organising the food, but you needn't announce it with trumpets to all and sundry. If you are just 'being careful' with what you eat, then for the ultimate enjoyment for all, heed this advice:

"Sorry, I don't eat that", rather than "I can't eat that". Phrasing is everything—saying it this way exhibits a sense of decisiveness and power over how you nourish your body rather than sounding as if you have relinquished control to an oppressive outside source. It'll mean people are less likely to inquire about the reason you can't or won't eat something. Be whimsical and throwaway in your comment rather than aggressive. Inquiries of a delicate, medical and personal nature are discourteous, and so, *polite* company will probe no further.

Bring your own. If you are in a casual lunch setting, in an office or in attendance where someone hasn't explicitly prepared a meal for you, then bring what *you* want to eat to the party. If they ask why just say swiftly and in a matter-of fact tone, "I'm on a restricted diet for medical reasons" . Again, a conversation that can go no further without feeling impolite. Refrain from adding emotion when delivering your response to questions, in fact be a little curt. It may be a white lie, but be honest to yourself. You *are* dieting for medical reasons, to gain better health! Just make sure the food you do bring is relatively healthy and is a passable excuse.

Serve yourself where possible. Learn proper portion control and exert conservative restraint over what goes on your plate. Half of the plate should be made up of whole-foods (as they came from the earth) such as salad or vegetables in a variety of colours, it's no use if they are smothered in cheese or creamy dressings—that defeats the purpose. A quarter of the plate, or around the size of your palm, should be protein (meat if you are that way inclined) or complex carbohydrates such as legumes, beans or lentils. The last quarter to be made up of the 'extras' which are manufactured foods such as bread, cheese, or pastry. Any healthy fats or dressings such as nuts, olive oil, dressings, or butter should measure in volume to about the size of your thumb for one serving.

Leave something on your plate. Food culture and dining etiquette varies the world over. In the UK it is considered rude not to finish a certain dish and then continue to further courses. Leaving vast portions on your plate is a sign of displeasure. If you wish to decline pudding, make sure you have a little food remaining on your plate. It is a visual cue that you are satisfied and have been fed enough in previous courses. If you do clear your plate, be honest about whether you would like pudding or not. It is not considered rude to decline the third course, but as a whole, your fellow guests, host or waiter will be most puzzled and ask "if you are sure" several times. It is not very often you see an Englishman resist a sticky toffee pudding at a dinner party, despite how full he may be. It is his duty to please his hostess with compliments on her great cooking. We all secretly size each other up by our ability to dish out great English classics and compare them to our personal matriarch's recipes. If an Englishman *has* stuffed himself to the rafters, what you won't see are his spartan choices for the next few days of simple sandwiches and apples and a brisk country walk to make up for the over indulgence. It's as much about balance, as it is to gear himself up and make space for the next round of dinner parties and social events.

Zip it to zip it. If your diet becomes more about fad than lifestyle and health, then you have the balance wrong. If you talk about the subject incessantly it quickly becomes tiring for all involved, and a wide open target for sabotage. People are more likely to understand *why* you are dieting if you are trying to increase fertility, staving off the onset of diabetes, or insulin resistance, lowering cholesterol or reducing your sugar and salt intake. If you are dieting for vanity's sake and tell all, then out come the "but you look fine" comments and puzzled expressions. When you claim you are trying to slim into an outfit (or perhaps old outfits), be aware that people may subconsciously try to sabotage you. They don't mean to, and even do so unknowingly, it's a subconscious thing that humans do. Be one step ahead and keep quiet about your plans and goals. Do it in secret and wow them with the outcome.

Eating for pleasure

One of the key areas for self mastery concerning food is learning how to eat for pleasure. One might think that this is a dangerous slope towards gluttony, but it is in fact quite the opposite. We are *more* likely to overeat when we under appreciate the food that is in front of us. This is the reason why, when faced with a box of cheap chocolate we are able to mindlessly eat the lot then end up staring into the bottom of the box wondering what on earth happened. I should like to challenge you to do the same with a beautifully presented box of decadent chocolate with a high amount of cocoa. It cannot be done without making one feel rather nauseous. When you take notice of your food and know the story behind it, even if it just came from the 'luxury' section of the supermarket, you associate that food with a higher sense of importance and therefore treat it with a little more respect and appreciation.

If we take this modest but luxury mindset with all foods, then nothing should ever be considered 'forbidden', and from there we can rebuild our relationship with food. For instance you might adore crumpets for breakfast slathered in anything sweet. Saturday mornings are now your 'crumpet morning' and something as a family you all look forward to. It starts the weekend off with some feel-good factor and stops you from eating crumpets or toast plus all that delicious sugar you might slather on it through the week. This mindset makes it much easier to make healthy choices for breakfast in the week as you know that you aren't being *kept* from eating what you want, as you have made a deliberate choice for the best *time* and place to enjoy it completely.

Learning to eat for pleasure cannot be achieved without first raising your standards. This means refraining from eating 'on the go' where possible, and *treating* yourself to the *experience* of eating. Refinement means choosing to slow down in this fast paced society. To be mindful, purposeful and poised. It means choosing to sit quietly to enjoy your afternoon cup of tea, or savouring your dinner at a beautifully dressed table. Pleasure seeking, coupled with the act of eating will not only allow your body the time to assimilate nourishing itself, but the entire act of it becomes something to associate with pleasure and rest. Once you capture the art of this you won't want to let it go. There have been books written by women of other nations regarding weight loss, the core messages simply advocate slowing down to eat and choosing the *best* quality possible. It's not really all that hard to get to grips with. Consuming fast food at a fast pace not only lends itself to poor digestion and mindlessness but on many an occasion, poor manners too. Be kind to yourself and raise the bar.

Exercise without knowing it

Now granted, there have always been people throughout the history of time who have been what we would consider to be 'overweight', but the statistics don't lie. Our modern culture is a hot-bed of obesity. It is purely down to what you *choose* to fill your stomach with, and how little you leave your house. Televisions, corner shops, computers and the like do little to inspire us to venture far from, or entertain ourselves outside of the home.

Sweating for sweating's sake is a modern preoccupation and we have been made to feel it is necessary in order to be 'healthy', when in fact our bodies are built to be healthy, naturally. It is only down to our over consumption of modern convenience foods, coupled with our sedentary and largely indoor lifestyles that force our chubby bottoms shame faced into the gym, or back onto the sofa through sheer feelings of hopelessness. It's no use telling you that spending hours on a treadmill will make you healthy/beautiful/happier because if you aren't already doing it willingly and *enjoying it*, then there is little chance of you adopting a new lifestyle centred around 'fitness for fitness sake'. Going to the gym or timetabled fitness classes out of guilt or pressure to 'train' isn't what someone inclined to live a life of refinement would do. We don't bow down to societal pressure, but we can choose to do *something* about our health in ways that **enrich us as a whole person.**

The way in which you can approach exercise in on old-time English way is to make use of the beautiful countryside and shoehorn cultural hobbies into your daily life that require leaving the house.

Here are some ways in which you can be inspired by our green and pleasant land in order to perk up that bottom without even knowing it:

- Walk instead of taking the car for short journeys to the shops and the school run. Oh yes, that means even in the rain. Investing in a good pair of wellingtons and a mackintosh will see you through decades of downpours.
- Abandon the supermarket. Find you nearest grocer, butcher and baker and visit them once or twice a week (on foot) for fresh local produce. They are usually in town, so grab a wicker basket and make a stroll of it.
- Build a weekend walk into your family traditions. Research routes and places of interest to couple with a spot of exercise as well as education and enrichment. Or join a local rambling club if the family aren't interested.
- Find a sport you love and join a local team. The socialising and camaraderie will make you forget you are exercising at all. Good sports for this balance are Tennis and Cricket, the social life involved make it a bonus.

- Go riding. Horses of course, or if you like, a bicycle. Both are great exercise but give back in a way that stomping on a treadmill never will.

- Grow your own veg or garden. You don't need much space for a few pots if you are lacking acreage. Feeling the fresh air and having some sun on your face *is* considered exercise compared to sitting on the sofa.

- Explore local history. Treat yourself to a membership to heritage organisations. Make a picnic and get out of the house to visit historic places and gardens as often as possible. Many have parkland to explore.

- Never feel guilty for 'relaxing', just make sure you spend at least 70% of the time *exercising the mind* while the body relaxes. Read, puzzle, or watch factual television on the landscape of England's green and pleasant land. Take notes and explore it on foot next week.

- Lastly, the greatest of all English suggestions; adopt a dog. It will need walking and you'll have no excuse not to get your daily exercise, come rain or shine.

OLD HATS & DIRTY LINEN

A CLASSIC ENGLISH WARDROBE & RULES OF DRESS

It's hardly news to us that impressions and judgments are made upon first meeting. Though we believe more care should be taken towards refining ones manners and affability, it is still important that the wardrobe also plays a part in letting your new acquaintance know a few key things about you. The first clue being whether you are concerned with behaving and dressing appropriately according to the environment you find yourself in. Obvious rebellion and lack of consideration for others is clear with a man baring his chest in a supermarket, or a woman in a skirt so short or top so low it flashes the unsuspecting. Consider also the parent who takes their child to school while wearing pyjamas, or the guest who wears white to a wedding. Apparent poor manners aside, there are rules in English society about what to wear and when, for not only highly formal occasions but also in the street on a daily basis. Not everyone can be highly fashionable and afford couture, but we can all be appropriate and good mannered in our rules of dress. Our adherence to one of the very basic of social codes demonstrates that we are willing to please, are considerate of others, and have respect for the society that surrounds us.

Forget the idea that to be considered upper crust you must have a wardrobe hot off the runway or need to be in 'full dress' at all times. Nay, the true English lady and gentleman dresses not in a way to rival movie stars or panders to the fashion elitists. Instead they buy to keep, and they buy for comfort and practicality. An intelligent approach to dressing is to buy in order to *re-wear*. The English are not ashamed to be seen in the same clothes, and they prefer to buy classics that can easily be transformed with accessories or jewellery. If you study it closely, the English adhere to an unwritten code of uniform adopted by many who care more for enjoyable experiences in life than parading about, and they definitely enjoy getting more for their money than flashing the cash on fast fashion.

The classic old-time English prefer to dress in a manner that is timeless. If one has been unfortunate and not inherited most of their wardrobe from their mother or father, he goes out to emulate and collect pieces for a classic English wardrobe of his own accord. This is done slowly, over time, and with much consideration for quality, and appealing to their peers in a way that does not make them stand out. The Englishman prefers instead to blend in to the quiet, restrained, but beautifully refined circle to which he belongs.

If you wish to have a wardrobe full of pieces that give you joy and make you feel good every time you wear them, and have something to don for every occasion, you must first evaluate your attitude towards clothes and how you relate to the idea of quality over quantity. We are living in a society that embraces a throw away culture of most consumer goods, and nowhere is this more apparent than in the fashion industry. This is what we need to turn from, embracing an old way of thinking and purchasing items.

In fact if you want to be truly English, you must forget the very *idea* of being fashionable and instead aim to be refined in taste, to look timeless, and always appropriate. There have been exceptions to the rules; case in point the Duke of Windsor, who was very keen on fashion and fame, but those trappings helped him fall from his pedestal rather swiftly.

Choose classic and conservative over fashionable and flippant

As a resident of a civilised democratic nation you have a voice. With every purchase, you are voting with your pound for the practices and retail experience you support and desire more of. Every time you swipe you credit card at a fast fashion retail store you are essentially passing a vote that poor quality and cheap labour are something you support. Thus the coffers of that conglomerate are further filled to enable them to churn out more items destined for landfill within a season or two. This throwaway culture is not only damaging our planet beyond belief, it is lowering the consumer/producer standards of our entire society. If you are lucky enough to afford to clothe yourself, you should be making considered purchases for your wardrobe, as you would a motor vehicle. A sensible and conservative approach towards buying clothes is easily compared to all major purchase considerations and looks much like this:

Brand and heritage

Ask yourself if you support the brand and if you have a mutually positive relationship. Are they trustworthy, transparent, and concerned with quality, or do they want to sell you cheap items in vast quantity? Are the two-for-one offers seemingly irresistible, even though you only went in for one item? Consider the sales team, are they miserable, uncaring, and too young to be confident enough to look you in the eye, let alone advise you? Is the attention of the staff merely on stock replenishment, readily taking your cash, and watching out for shoplifters? Or are they welcoming, attentive, and really know the product? The busyness of a store will also give you an indication of how people spend their money there. It is generally fast and without care? A crowded shop with items sloppily piled high or hanging precariously on stuffed rails does not scream quality, in item or experience. There is no shame in making a choice to spend your hard earned money in a store that makes you feel good. Just because we all need to clothe our naked bodies doesn't mean we should settle for the cheapest option possible. Your image and the personal brand you project are reflected in the quality of clothing you select. Nothing makes you feel nicer than buying a beautiful item from a store that practices mutual respect, openly appreciates you, and values your custom. Remember, when you look good, you feel good, and those feelings can be woven into the purchase experience as much as the threads of the garment itself.

Build quality

Is the construction and finish of the item sound? Poorly finished garments will have loose threads, wobbly seams, and uneven hemlines. The inside of the garment matters as much as the outside and is ultimately what keeps it all together. Make sure to also look for stains, pulls, and easy creasing—if it looks poor quality or is damaged in the store, it won't look any better at home, even if you think you can fix it. Remember, if it has been put on the sale rack *because* of this condition it is *not* a bargain. All you are doing is buying a defective item. Just because it's *cheaper* doesn't make it a valuable item to you, in fact probably less so as you will mentally associate it as being 'broken' or less-than.

Materials used

Feel the garment, does the fabric feel rough, shiny, or cheap? Or does it feel luxurious, nice to the touch, and high quality? If it doesn't feel good upon immediate first impression, it won't feel nice on. Thinner materials will wear quicker especially on hard wearing areas such as elbows, knees, and bottoms. Poor quality fabrics will not launder well in the long run. They are particularly susceptible to over-shrinking and the seam alignments warping once washed. Opt for natural materials such as 100% cotton, wool, linen, silk, and leather where possible. Not only will they look and feel better when you wear them but they will stand the test of time, giving you better value for money.

Maintenance requirements

The majority of modern clothing is now made to withstand machine washing, or at the very least a hand washing or dry cleaning. Always take note of the garment care instructions before purchasing an item and consider whether you are able, and more importantly willing, to provide the garment with the attention it needs. Note that cashmere, silks, and wools have very specific care instructions for laundering and also require special storage. Consider your investment of not only money but time. When you take good care of your clothing it will last and maintain a fresher appearance for much longer.

Mileage

Is the garment really only fashionable *right now,* and could be considered a throwaway piece? If so, contemplate very carefully your budget for such items. Buying 'wear once' items is not a sound investment and costs money you could put towards something you will enjoy wearing again and again. Look for classics that will remain in your wardrobe for many years. You should aim to spend the larger portion of any clothing budget on items of superior quality to ensure they last through the seasons and provide the best mileage for your investment. It's no use buying cheaper alternatives of classic items that you intend to wear for years to come, only to have them fall apart after the first few wears. What you put in, you get out.

Test drive

Always, always try a garment on before purchasing. If you ordered an item online make sure to keep the tags intact and keep hold of the packing materials in case you need to return it. When shopping and trying items consider these tactics in order to have the best experience possible:

- Freshen up. Not only is it good manners to be clean and well presented, but you will feel better about yourself in the changing room. Going in unwashed, unshaven and with mismatched underwear is never going to make you feel wonderful, no matter how stunning the suit or dress.

- Neither try nor buy clothing on a completely empty stomach, or immediately after eating. Especially not after a boozy lunch. You want to be sober of mind, not hungry, and certainly not bloated and uncomfortable.

- Take a good look at the cut of the garment and try your usual size as well as a size up or a size down depending on the pattern shapes. If billowy and loose, consider the next size down. If the item will show a little skin, try a size up. The size on the label is absolutely no reflection on the value of your body and you will always look a million times better in an item that fits well, regardless of what the hanger size says. Manufacturer sizing standards are always poles apart from one shop to the next, so it pays to ignore any anxiety associated with 'size' and see it for what it is. As simple as picking out whether blue or red looks better on you, the same goes for the mark on the label. Buy what looks better, not the size you *wish* you could be wearing. If it bothers you that much, once purchased and taken home carefully blot out the number on the label with a permanent marker or cut out the label entirely and move on to better things in your beautifully fitting clothes.

- Take your time and never shop when you are rushed. You might make decisions you regret and could potentially miss the window to return items.
- If you are considering making an expensive purchase that you hadn't planned, it pays to delay the satisfaction and ask the store if they'd be willing to hold the item for you for 24 hours. If after that time you are still in love with the item and absolutely have to have it, then buy it. This separates the emotion from the experience and saves your pennies when you realise you don't really need that extra handbag or suit after all.

Empire over imports

The British clothing industry is alive and well. It has always been fastidious and reliable, it just doesn't shout from the rooftops like major brands. Restrained but reliable and terribly English, some British clothing companies have been in business now for hundreds of years. The old time English have always remained loyal to clothiers and outfitters who provide quality British-made items. It feels good to support a homegrown business that provide not only a wonderful service but beautiful products too.

Despite the flood of imports from the Far East, many are now turning away from over-consumption of fast fashion. They are looking for ethically made 'slow' products and clothing produced right here in Great Britain. The benefit of choosing to buy British is that the products are generally designed for our specific lifestyle, and obviously with consideration of the weather. It is of the utmost importance that designers have a deep understanding of the way in which we live in this country. A wardrobe filled with light fabrics suitable for only the nicest of Californian weather, aside from looking ridiculous here, will not keep you warm come the British winter. Our two weeks of summer are little catered for, but choices are abundant for our remaining seasons, and they are designed to last.

English gentlemen in particular shop where their father shopped, and his father before him. Many pieces returning time and time again to the original workshop for general upkeep and alteration. This fosters a relationship between the outfitter and the gentleman which can never be emulated on the general high street. On the more expensive side it may be, but one good suit can last for decades, with many men wearing suits their father once owned himself. Such is the timelessness, quality, and longevity of the product. As a female, I'm the first to express my jealousy at the options available in England for our men. It is rare to find an equivalent to Jermyn Street for ladies, however there are some wonderful heritage brands producing beautiful items for both sexes if you take the time to seek them out.

If you would like to support the coffers of Great Britain and buy traditionally elegant pieces for your wardrobe, look for companies granted with the Royal Warrant. Holders of this prestigious status are listed in an online directory. There you will find manufacturers of most all items for the wardrobe, from socks to hats, suiting to hair combs. Companies cannot apply for a Royal Warrant unless they have been supplying the households of HM The Queen, HRH The Duke of Edinburgh, or HRH The Prince of Wales for at least five years out of the last seven. Standards must be high and the company is thoroughly vetted during the process of obtaining a warrant. Though not all companies listed are British, the vast majority are, and many have been trading for at least a hundred years. Choosing to purchase from these companies not only supports the practices of economic self-sufficiency and supply, but buys you a little slice of the royal lifestyle.

A classic wardrobe and its association with the English lifestyle

It would appear that in modern times many have forgotten how to dress, not only literally, but emotionally and economically too. With the advent of an overwhelming amount of choices we have become blind to what suits us in favour of what is fashionable, and we largely dress according to what other people expect of us. Sometimes we dress to provoke, to show disrespect as an act of rebellion. At no age is this turbulence more obvious than with young men and women in their first flush of adulthood. The pressure to dress to be considered 'cool' in the teenage years will bring about a cultural uniform according to what is trendy at the time, yet when those individuals grow up, so used to conformity after years of school and tribe-uniform they never really learn how to dress appropriately or shop well.

We shan't pretend that the older we get the less we care to look nice, or care less about what other people think, but the pendulum tends to sway a little further into the ideals of comfort and quality. This desire for comfort lies dangerously close to the "jeans are suitable for all occasions" mindset to which so many middle aged people have fallen prey to. Thankfully the Englishman's uniform lends itself perfectly to comfort and ease of choice, while upholding a sense of pride in one's appearance and managing to look pulled together. You will have noted earlier in this lesson that we should be moving *further* away from fashion and trends and closer to simplicity and enduring style. Here lies below the steps, tips and pieces required for collecting a *classic* English wardrobe that will suit your lifestyle twenty years from now, as much as it does today. If you buy well, those pieces will long remain with you too.

High street stores are selling what is in vogue *now*, but *we* are concerned with what will still be stylish in five, ten, or even fifty years time. It takes a lifetime to mindfully curate and shop for such a thing as the 'complete wardrobe' but if you indulge yourself in learning about the heritage of the tailors, makers, and cobblers who will outfit you for the years you have left, your relationship to the garments that clothe you will be that much more special. Dressing well gives you a confidence and self-assurance that no on-trend item ever will. 'Things' will not bring you happiness, but things that bring out your quiet confidence and help you to feel at ease in life and always appropriate will certainly help.

The foolish man buys his clothes to wear and enjoy but for a season, the Englishman buys his clothes to live in and enjoy for a lifetime.

AN ENGLISH GENTLEMAN'S WARDROBE

There was a time when gentlemen knew how to dress properly, or at least their valets did. Information and rules of dress passed from one generation to another. Sadly, in modern times the humble t-shirt, tracksuit, and football strip have done away with any sense of masculine elegance or appropriateness. If one has personal taste for a refined classic wardrobe, it is now an education to unearth all by ones self. Though ones wardrobe should be filled with pieces that uniquely reflect his style, there are certain design pieces, which, if invested in and collected with care ensure he maintains a wardrobe of classic items that will last through the years and perform well at any occasion.

This list is not exhaustive but showcases the best of classic English gentleman's style. Should you wish to add to your wardrobe, included below are suggestions of outfitters and places to source the best Great Britain has to offer. Most are Royal Warrant holders or, if from overseas have a strong heritage brand *synonymous* with the English lifestyle.

A classic gentleman's wardrobe

Weatherproofs

The iconic **Trench Coat** was a design brought to the fore by officers of the First World War. Worn in the trenches, traditionally it is made of cotton gabardine, a lightweight but breathable waterproof fabric, and is a good option for an inclement, often changeable climate. It is suggested to purchase loose enough to wear over a suit. The classic design of a trench or 'mac' includes a double breasted ten button closure, epaulettes, raglan sleeves, a storm and gun flap, and is belted at the waist. A traditional length is below the knee to mid-calf and usually khaki or camel in colour. Many menswear designers have tried to replicate the look, but fail to hit the mark on true durability or weatherproofing. This overcoat is meant to protect you from the rain, and should you wish to purchase one, aim to seek a classic design from a long-standing, trusted manufacturer. It is continually argued as to who invented the original trench coat, however reliable companies to source from are Aquascutum or Burberry, both noted for their loyalty to the original design and superior finishes.

A classic **Waxed Jacket** is synonymous with English country living. Makers of the finest are the unrivalled J. Barbour & Sons. For dog walking, shooting, or outdoor pursuits, no country gent's wardrobe is complete without one. Ignore the company's recent diversion toward dressing the 'trendy crowd' and source yours from a specialised country clothing outfitters who will supply original styles suitable for country wear. The classic Beaufort and Bedale models are worth looking at, both are weather and thorn proof. A well cared for waxed Barbour will last you a lifetime if you maintain it. Rewaxing once a year will keep it in good order. Barbour also offer a rewax, repair, and alteration service for a nominal fee should you require it.

A **Wax Cap** is great for casual country wear and inclement weather.

The **Umbrella** is a necessary accessory for most of us, the classic choice usually being a crooked handled design and in walking length for the gentlemen. While sporting and golf umbrellas come in handy in a bind, nothing complements a gentleman's ensemble better than a classically styled model. Especially when out for the evening or attending formal events, a sophisticated umbrella finishes the whole look. Prices and designs can vary, but a restrained navy or black with mock-horn or wooden crooked handle is a sensible choice. Modern automatic umbrellas make operating a breeze. Bear in mind however that the purchase of a good umbrella brings with it the responsibility to remember to not only take it with you, but return home with it also. A task easier said than done! Country gentlemen can choose a golf umbrella, most sourced from country outfitters and brands synonymous with the lifestyle. Though note that golf umbrellas are usually styled and manufactured for advertising rather than longevity and practicality. Acquire yours from Fulton, umbrella suppliers to the Queen, or if you are feeling like treating yourself, head to James Smith & Sons (go in person for the experience). If one is feeling particularly flamboyant in style and budget try Pasotti online.

Suppliers: Fulton, James Smith & Sons, Pasotti, Dubarry, Schöffel.

Wellington Boots, popularised by Arthur Wellesley, the first Duke of Wellington, became a staple of practical footwear for the English since the early nineteenth century. Ideal for country weekends, dog walking, sporting events, agricultural work, and all manner of menial daily pursuits such as garden maintenance and popping to the shops—these puddle avoiders are most delightful to wear. Pretenders come and go, but a classic 'British Racing Green' pair from Hunter cannot be beaten for staving off 'mizzle', drizzle, or heavy downpours. Welly liners or shooting socks to line the boot are optional, just make sure to tuck your trousers in to avoid looking foolish. The very point of wearing wellingtons is to avoid getting wet or muddy, *not* to look cool. Store them properly on a rack (upside down) or boot tray to avoid upsetting the lady of the house, and *always* check for marauding mice and spiders before pulling on a boot—both a bitter experience one does not forget in a hurry.

Suppliers: Barbour, Hunter, Orvis, Le Chameau, Dubarry.

Overcoats and outerwear

The original **Car Coat** is simply cut, single breasted, mid thigh length, and cut of wool, cashmere, and in some cases tweeds. Invented in the early 1900s to protect driver and passenger alike from the elements, before the advent of the windshield, roof and heating, it has been a staple in the gentleman's wardrobe ever since. As the development of the motorcar moved on, car coats have since been adapted for the modern lifestyle and manufactured in lighter materials such as shower-proof cottons and linens. Car coats are a stylish alternative to the longer length macintosh or heavy winter wool overcoat and make a classic inter-seasonal option for professional and casual wear. Keep colours muted in navy, khaki, or camel and your materials weatherproof for longevity and practicality. Conservative simplistic designs with welted pockets and hidden button plackets lend themselves well to professional wear over suits. While zippered or exposed closures and informal patch pocket designs are better suited to off duty days.

Suppliers: Orvis, Burberry, Samuel Windsor.

The **Sport Jacket** is a design akin to a blazer, but intended to be worn without matching trousers and often looser or 'sack like' in cut with little or no shaping to the waist. Cuts and designs are generally more relaxed and fabrics which wear well are chosen such as corduroy, suede tweed, wools, and for summer wear, stonewashed cottons, linens, and seersuckers. A relaxed cousin to the more formal blazer, the sport coat is single or double vented, and features a single breasted one, two or three button closure, narrow lapels, and a breast pocket. Patch pockets are also often seen. A common design feature are leather elbow patches on tweeds, corduroys, and wools. They are a hard-working favourite among university lecturers and intellectuals alike. Wear with chinos, jeans or moleskin trousers and over an Oxford shirt or fair isle for smart casual wear.

Suppliers: Hawes & Curtis, Brook Taverner, Charles Tyrwhitt, Peter Hahn.

The **Formal Blazer**, with design features inspired by military uniforms are worn for semi-formal and formal occasions. Often in dark navy or black suiting, or new wool, with gold breast and cuff buttons in a single or double breasted finish, vented with one to three button closure. Breast pockets feature as well as padding to the shoulder. The intention is to look sharp. The cut of the jacket is a personal choice with some favouring a straight classic Oxford fit (most traditional) while fitter men opt for a 'fashion fit' from chest to hip. Blazers in suiting or velvet fabrics are traditionally worn with formal cut trousers in suiting or wool. Chinos are permissible so long as the shoe and the event remains semi-formal. For the velvet 'smoking' blazer, self-covered buttons are used along with satin finishing, and sometimes frogging—it is not to be worn before dusk.

Suppliers: Richard James, Charles Tyrwhitt, Brook Taverner, Gant, Cordings of Piccadilly.

The **Bomber, Field, or Flight Jacket** are styles to be worn on casual occasions. Bomber and flight styles reflecting the heritage of Great Britain and once again taking inspiration from the practical utility restraint that won them favour with our RAF squadrons in WW2. All styles are cropped to hip length, zipped, loose in style and form, collared and deep pocketed. Some fitted with a buckle at the waist. Ribbing is also used at the waist line and cuffs offering protection from cold breezes. Modern styles are manufactured in man made fabrics but classic styles are shearling, suedes, and leathers. The 'Field Jacket' features a lighter design with usually four patch pockets and button closures. Fabrics are cotton drills, leather, chambray, or man made shower proof materials.

Suppliers: Aviation Leathercraft, Orvis, Charles Tyrwhitt, Filson.

The **Raincoat** is the Englishman's loyal friend. Ever needed and most valued, the raincoat has many guises and styles, the most refined being a classic overcoat style with minimal embellishment helping to avoid the collection of water in external seams or stitch work. Lengths vary from just above the knee to ankle length, many including a storm flap, fly front and adjustable buckle sleeves. Designs are usually lightweight allowing the coat to be removed and carried easily in the crook of the arm or folded neatly to be stored in the car. Waxed raincoats are common but do often emit a rather persistent damp doggy smell seemingly favoured by the country set. These waxed styles are oft worn with wellington or country boots. Town dwellers should choose navy, black, or camel, fly front, mid length designs which not only complements a formal work outfit, but helps them to stay dry during the commute in and out of the city. Cagoules are an altogether different animal and are used in the most fervent of rainstorms, generally when hiking, touring, or on other casual weekend pursuits.

Suppliers: *Aquascutum, Jermyn Street Outfitters, Brook Taverner, Moss Bros, Charles Tyrwhitt.*

The **Overcoat** is a generic term for all styles of 'topcoat' garment, but here we refer to it as a single or double breasted, often cashmere or heavy wool coat to be worn on smart occasions. Tweeds and wide herringbones provide a casual weekend and sporting alternative, both claiming a wide variety of lapel options, some formal choices are styled with velvet. The classic overcoat, knee length or longer with flap or jetted pockets, and a notched lapel is a supremely elegant and classic staple in the gentleman's wardrobe. Perfect to lend warmth over a suit or jacket, the overcoats design has remained largely conservative, and while known by many names, the cut has remained consistent since its origins in the mid 1800s when the flamboyant regency styles took a turn towards the less decorative victorian aesthetic. Before this time gentlemen wore what were known as body coats, to be worn inside as well as outside (and never removed in public) while the invention of the larger and looser over coat, providing no waist seam, added another layer to be worn atop a jacket for outdoor wear only. The classic colour for the overcoat is a plain black or charcoal to ensure its versatility in pairing other items from the wardrobe. Camel toned overcoats are also favoured for leisure wear and a less formal look, often coupled with a fur or shearling collar. Note also the **Covert Coat**, originating as an equestrian jacket, it features a style similar in design to the overcoat but is shorter in length and features a poaching pocket. This style is much favoured by gentlemen of the hunting, racing, and country scene.

Suppliers: *Jermyn Street Outfitters, Austin Reed, Jaeger, Hawes & Curtis, Charles Tyrwhitt.*

The **Quilted Jacket & Gilet** are the reserve of the country set, or those on the water, or whose pursuits include horses, dog walking, sailing, and general country life. They have recently found favour among those in town for their lightweight yet classic styling and is a good all-season option for drier but chilly days. Worn in casual settings, choose yours in a classic navy, moss, or evergreen. Most quilted jackets and vests are down filled, some options may be fleece or flannel lined. Choose one with a thicker polyester outer fabric to avoid sprouting feathers where possible. Funnel necks, zipped closures, and press-stud button flaps are common as well as patch and interior pockets. Choose yours to fit slimline without waist gathers to layer under larger raincoats for added warmth, or bigger to wear over sweaters and a polo or rugby shirt. The famous fleece Lyndon II gilet from Schöffel is a classic and stylish option for layering over Tattersall shirts or light sweaters and has been long-favoured with British agricultural and farming communities for the warmth and utility it provides.

Suppliers: Barbour, Crew Clothing, Dubarry, Gant, Orvis, Schöffel.

Headwear

Sadly, for hats to make an appearance on the crown of a gentlemen today, the bells of the local church must ring or toll, weather needs to be below freezing, or have the British Isles experience a heatwave—the latter being the most unlikely. Gone are the days of the hat featuring in a gentleman's daily outfit and with its decline, so much charm, etiquette, and sartorial flair is all but lost. The standard issue beanie and the branded baseball cap do not count as stylish headwear to the English gentleman, both being the very last option he should take when looking to shield his crown from rain or shine.

Should a modern gentleman wish to return to a graceful existence and don a daily chapeau, there are many options for him but most require the wearing of a formal outfit for it not to look out of place. That being said, even a casual hat can add gravitas to an outfit. Here we shall explore the more casual and semi-formal options for headwear, what to wear with them, and where:

The **Flat Cap** is an essential in the country gent's wardrobe. Offering smart casual headwear from walking the dog to tinkering in the garage, the flat cap and baker boy are also worn for shooting. The tweed or flannel 'Newsboy' being a wider option, or a 'Highland Hat' makes a popular choice styled similar to a deerstalker, but lighter in frame.

Suppliers: Farlows, A Hume, Orvis, Schöffel.

The **Waxed Bushman, or Felt Hat** is a good country life, sporting, or walking option. With shape and style akin to the Panama, pair this autumn/winter style with wax jackets, quilted gilets, and casual half-zip sweaters. Traditionally constructed on a wooden block, felt hats are sometimes finished with leather strap and feather, and even gun cartridge detailing, offering a stylish finish to a country look. The Bushman is the same shape as the wider brimmed felt hat, often in weatherproofed waxed cotton or leather.

Suppliers: A Hume, The House of Bruar, Christy's of London, Lock & Co Hatters.

A cotton **Cricket or Baseball Cap** is suitable for garden work, DIY and very casual events. Not to be worn to work or at a social event that offered more than a last minute invitation. Too many have fallen into the honey trap of this 'easy option'. Casual but boring, and never smart, the cotton cap should be reserved for all but home, when working out, or when actually playing cricket on a village green.

Suppliers: Village Hats, or your local car dealership, and tourist market stalls.

For the height of summer a **Straw Fedora, Boater, or Panama** are stylish and flexible options. They are extremely versatile according to your chosen outfit. Looking equally smart with light summer suits or shirt sleeves and more casual with a polo and shorts. Choose genuine handwoven Panamas from Ecuador. The 'Montechristi' model being the most exclusive and luxurious, some taking up to four months to weave. Some straw summer hats can be rolled making them ideal for travel. The Planter Panama is an elegant and distinctive style with a round flat brim and changeable brim bands, most synonymous with sugar plantation workers and river boatmen on the Mississippi. Not distinctly English, but a good option for sun protection saving one from resorting to less stylish options. The **Classic Boater** (or Skimmer), crafted from stiff sisal straw and topped with a band of Petersham ribbon offers a traditionally English summer look perfect for picnics and barbecues. Often favoured by gentlemen attending semi-formal waterside events such as the Henley Royal Regatta, they are particularly fetching coupled with linen or seersucker jackets and bold striped boating blazers.

Suppliers: The Panama Hat Company, Christy's of London, Lock & Co Hatters.

Heavier winter options for freezing and snowy conditions include thick **Astrakhan and Cossack** hats, made famous by the Soviets. Fashioned from a distinctive looped and curled wool, or often fur, they are brimless with a wide upturn on the forehead, fit close to the head and fold flat when not worn. They look striking when worn with city business attire and woollen or cashmere overcoats. **Trappers, Stalkers, Ushanka** (*trans:* ear flap hat) **and Deerstalkers** with fleece or faux fur linings and 'ears' that fold up and away when not in use are favourable for sub-zero temperatures and should be coupled with weekend casual and sporting attire. The knitted **Wool Beanie, Skull/Stocking Cap or Watch Cap** (oft worn by fisherman and fictional burglars) is another casual option for cold and inclement weather, but should not be worn in the working week by gentleman in white collar industries if he wishes to retain a smart business appropriate appearance. All winter hat options should be black, navy, grey or in the natural colour of fur or fleece as one does not want to be mistaken for a winter sportsman or search and rescue operative.

Suppliers: Lock & Co Hatters, Christy's of London, Bates Gentleman's Hatters, Country Attire Outfitters.

For smarter town and business-commuter wear, a gentleman wearing a formal business suit may choose to wear a narrower brimmed wool or fur felt **Trilby, Homburg, or Fedora** in city appropriate colours such as black, grey, or navy. For the truly bold, an **English Bowler** is both smart and an incredible talking piece now so rarely seen. Originally created in 1850 as a hard hat to protect gamekeepers while horse riding on patrols (higher crowned top hats were often knocked off by low branches), the look has become synonymous with the English lifestyle, but do pair this with your smartest attire only. Match the fabrics of your hats as closely as possible to the fabrics of your outwear; heavier fabric hats such as tweed, wool, and felt with wool or cashmere. Lighter cottons, linens, and straw better matched to summer suiting.

Hat care:

- Where possible, keep original hat boxes for storage.
- A felt or wool brush is a good investment to keep formal hats looking fresh and free of dirt and debris, brush them lightly after each use and air them for a few hours before returning to storage.
- Rest your hats gently on the brim, with tissue stuffed in the crown to keep its shape.
- Never store a hat for long periods on a stand, hook, or stacked atop another hat.
- Return your hat to your milliner for repair and reshaping if necessary.
- Consider professionally weatherproofing wool and felt hats at a dry cleaners or with your hatter for optimum lifespan.
- Never return a hat to storage when damp.
- Store hats in a cool, dark, dry place. Fluctuations in temperature can wreak havoc with glues and cause misshapen crowns and brims.

Remember: When it comes to hats, no matter in the country or city, you must remove them when indoors, and it is always polite to remove your hat when conversing with a lady.

Shoes and footwear

The long rich history and booming industry of English shoemakers is alive and well. Though priced higher than your average mass-manufactured shoe, when well taken care of, a good pair can last a gentleman a decade or more. There are a handful of quality shoemakers and cobblers still operating today that have shod feet of the good and famous from generations past and continue to do so today. It is said that you can tell a lot about a man by the style of his shoes and the care he takes of them. With so few luxury accessories to demonstrate a gentleman's taste and refinement available to him, the shoe is a sound investment for not only uplifting the appearance but making sure he takes good care of his feet. High quality off-the-peg designs are accessible to all, but if you truly wish to experience the luxury of made to measure shoes, head to Tricker's to have a last made from your very own feet for fitted perfection. If it's good enough for royalty, then it's good enough for the English gentleman. You may need to acquire a small loan first as the cost is extraordinary, yet so is the experience.

Suppliers: Loake, Tricker's, Grenson, G.H. Bass & Co, Oliver Sweeney, Foster & Son.

Town shoes

The **Oxford Shoe** is the classic shoe of choice for almost all formal occasions from school to business wear, to weddings and funerals. The Oxford shoe is quite literally straight laced and formal, sitting very close to the foot, low on the ankle, a flat heel, and with very little embellishment or excessive styling. Fully laced black, brown, tan, and oxblood leathers with leather soles are most classic. Plain toe Oxfords are the most formal and should be the option chosen for weddings and black tie events, ideally slimmer cut in black patent leather. While cap-toe Oxfords can lend themselves to business and semi formal wear. Wingtips with broguing (perforations originally designed to drain away excess water) can also be found and are best suited to pairing with tweed suits. This most casual and wider toe-boxed Oxford can lean gently towards weekend wear and coupling with country colours and informal trouser fabrics such as moleskin, needlecord, and corduroy.

A **Double Monk Buckle Shoe** is often found crisply styled in plain or patent leather to complement a sharp suit, but can feature in suede with rubber soles for a casual air, which pair nicely with tweed and wool and sometimes summer suiting. Originally designed centuries ago as foot protection for Monks performing manual labour, the style went on to gain popularity during the more elaborate men's fashions of the seventeenth and eighteenth centuries. It fell away into obscurity until recently when a resurgence of classic styles came about and a hyper-smart town shoe offering an alternative to the Oxford was sought. Single strap 'monks' are also available as a pared back option suitable for less elaborate outfits and perhaps better for business wear should you not want to draw *too* much attention to your hooves. Double monks can feature toecaps, and wingtips. They are sometimes found in ankle boot varieties.

The **Derby** is better suited for pairing with jeans or chinos when you wish to look smart, but not overdone as can be the case when pairing weekend wear with an Oxford shoe. The differences between the Derby and Oxford are subtle, evidence proven in the open lacing system on a Derby making the overall styling looser and less formal. Derby shoes are commonly manufactured in leathers, scotch grain, and suedes often featuring a thicker rubber or crepe sole. The ideal look of the shoe is to appear rather robust and utilitarian.

Suppliers: Loake, Tricker's, Grenson, Oliver Sweeney, Foster & Son.

Country, casual, and sporting shoes

The heavier Derby or **Brogue** with less formal and free-movement lacing is best suited for country wear. Many have heavily embossed soles in rubber or crepe for greater grip on the uneven, weather beaten surfaces of rural life. Rounded toes are appropriate for country wear, matching nicely with tweed, wool, moleskin, and casual jeans or chinos. Brogues are technically not in themselves a style of shoe, moreover a style of *decoration* on a shoe. With historically wet and boggy weather in the British Isles, men working outdoors would suffer soaked footwear. Styles evolved to include 'tooling' the leather with a brogue punch, creating small holes and perforations on a shoe in order to drain water off and promote quicker drying times. Broguing is usually reserved to the wingtip and sides on the shoe but fashion now dictates the location of the design, as opposed to function. Classically, the casual cousin to smarter shoes, Brogues are not thought to be appropriate after 6pm and *never* for black-tie, military, or celebratory events.

We credit the invention of the **Chelsea Boot** in 1837 to J. Sparkes-Hall, official boot maker to Queen Victoria. Designed to be worn and removed with minimal effort, the elastic-sided boot has remained popular ever since. Their streamlined classic looks lend themselves beautifully to tailored and casual looks. For more formal-minded gentlemen, the Chelsea boot is best reserved for semi-formal and casual wear. Instantly recognisable with their ankle-high fit and elastic sides, almond shaped toes are most popular. Narrow and pointed toe styles that lean towards a cowboy look are easily sourced, though these are strictly reserved for casual wear. The Chelsea boot is traditionally black leather but incarnations are made in dark brown and tan leathers for country wear. The Chelsea makes a good footwear option for wet and biting weather where wellingtons or hiking/snow boots may be inappropriate or seem over zealous. The method of ease of the elastic making the removal of dirty or wet boots when indoors even easier than laced boots.

Desert Boots are cousins of the higher ankled casual Chelsea boot but feature a cruder construction with unfinished edging, rough stitching, and open lacing as a closure method. Traditionally featuring a crepe rubber sole, with very simplistic upper construction from minimal pieces of leather or suede, and little visible stitching, this easy going style is best suited for wearing with jeans, heavy drill trousers, or chinos. Desert boots should be brown or sandy in colour but recent fashion houses are throwing all sorts of fabrics and printed patterns at the design in the name of 'fashion'. Never considered to be a business shoe they are best left to leisure wear only. Other originators and incarnations are Jodhpur and Chukka boots thought to originate from the footwear choice of Polo players not fancying the bother of long boots, with Chukkas worn by off duty army soldiers stationed in Burma and Cairo during the 1940s. The Desert boot gained worldwide popularity in the 1950s after manufacturer Clarks released their design which has ensured the brand name remains synonymous with the style.

Suppliers: Clarks, Chatham, Crockett & Jones, Herring Shoes, Loake, Tricker's.

The leather **Loafer**, originating from Norway in 1930 is a slip-on shoe that works well with many smart casual looks. Inspired by the Moccasin worn by native American Indians, the updated design was first worn by fishermen and farmers in Scandinavia. Now used for semi-formal and casual dressing, the slip-on is not generally considered suitable for business but can be paired with a suit for informal events. The Englishman would never consider wearing loafers without socks, which has become the trend of a younger European generation. Loafers in dark tan and oxblood are commonly paired with chino, moleskin, and corduroy trousers. Black if the trouser is of a darker shade. The loafer is versatile for town and casual wear. The looser styled **Moccasin or Driving Shoe** is similar in design but constructed in softer leathers and suedes, with all-in-one softer soles offering greater flexibility—reserved for casual and weekend wear only. Loafers are often embellished with a 'penny cut out' across the vamp, tassels, or horse-bits.

Suppliers: Tod's, G.H. Bass & Co, Russell & Bromley, Gucci.

Having slipped and fallen overboard from his boat on the Long Island Sound, Paul A. Sperry was intent on inventing a non-slip shoe to wear while sailing. Observing that his dog was able run over ice without slipping he took inspiration from his paws and used his knife to cut small ridges into the soles of rubber shoes much like the herringbone patterns seen in automobile tyres, and thus the traction **Boat/Deck Shoe** was born. Modelled with the upper construction of a casual hand-stitched Moccasin, with leather laces and mostly paired with non-marking rubber soles, the deck shoe has been popular footwear for sailors and skippers since its invention in 1935, and an approved choice of casual fair-weather footwear for the masses since the mid-twentieth century. Though not traditionally English, sailing as a sport around the British Isles and our rainy streets made this clever invention a go-to choice for leisure wear. Pair with, or go without socks, the choice is up to you but the Boat shoe is out of place in a corporate environment or when worn with anything other than jeans, chinos, or shorts. Common colours are dark brown and tan with lighter and duo-toned offerings for the adventurous.

Suppliers: Chatham, Sperry, Sebago.

Sandals, Mules and Flip-Flops are a comfortable choice for hot weather however there is much opinion and jokes proffered on the idea of sandals being an acceptable choice of footwear for the tasteful gentlemen. Some insist that they have no place in a man's wardrobe, while a youthful generation are turning to sandals for daily casual summer wear, even in town. The choice is yours, though really do consider if a deck shoe or sporty trainer would look better before slipping on a sandal. Sandals have absolutely no place in the boardroom or at a restaurant so your timing has to be impeccable if you wish to bare your feet to the world. We've heard it all regarding *socks and sandals*, if you must wear socks it makes sense to cover the rest of the foot with a shoe, lest you be the butt of the joke. Many types of sandals are available for vacation and beach wear, the most stylish options being a double-strap or muled Birkenstock. Followed by a walking sport-soled leather sandal with rip tape or buckle closures that encase the foot and back of the ankle. Leave the strappier sandals to the women as men rarely have aesthetically pleasing feet to expose so much, nor the delicacy of step or stride in which to comfortably keep them on the foot.

Suppliers: Birkenstock, Josef Seibel, Ecco, Charles Clinkard, Saltwater Sandals.

Trainers are meant for sportswear only, and no amount of hybridisation with tan leather or 'shoe like' styling will ever make the trainer suitable for formal events or the corporate environment. Leather trainers styled to look like

Derby shoes can look smart with cotton drill and chinos so long as the look is sleek and minimal with the sole erring on the thin side, but for a classically styled sports shoe they should be worn with shorts only. Many mainstream retailers are manufacturing semi-smart trainer shoes which hoodwink the younger generation into thinking they are business or date appropriate, but steer clear if you hope to wear them anywhere but the sports track, down the pub, running errands on the weekend, or around the home.

Suppliers: Clarks, Rieker, Skechers, Merrell.

Country Boots are essential for the Gentleman who resides in the country and are a suggested investment even for the visitor. Especially one who wishes to keep the polish on his shoes where it belongs. Ideal for dog walking, mucking out, and general splashing in puddles, the best styles are made from thick weather treated breathable leathers, sporting rubber soles and plenty of Gore-Tex lining. The best are made by Dubarry of Ireland offering traditional knee-high styling and robust construction as well as warmth. Wear with country appropriate clothing.

Suppliers: Dubarry of Ireland, Ariat, Rydale.

Suits

The Englishman will require four types of suit in his lifetime; a black suit, a dark navy or charcoal business suit, a lighter colour unlined linen or seersucker summer suit, plus a heavy winter Glen check, flannel, small houndstooth, tweed, or worsted wool suit for casual winter sporting events, weddings, or country wear. Ideally all types will come as a three piece, to enable the omitting of the waistcoat or jacket depending on formality. Specialist suits such as morning dress and the tuxedo can be hired unless one frequently attends weddings, black tie events, or is invited into royal enclosures. In which case it may be financially viable to invest in tailor made additions.

The wide array of fabrics, cuts, lapel options, breasted and button styling available are too vast to condense in these pages. So we defer to long established tailors who shall be able to guide a gentleman on what suit style and fabric will flatter him while remaining appropriate for the occasion he wishes to wear it. It pays to have your suits custom made, or at the very least professionally altered to provide that made to measure look.

Any English gentleman sourcing or commissioning a new suit should aim to look as conservative as possible, with a timeless, prestigious, and aristocratic air about him. Ideally avoiding all the trappings of suave, slim cuts, Italian styling, latest fashions and flatteries. He should aim to blend in to a line up of leading characters from incredibly English fantasy spy movies such as Kingsman and James Bond.

Some details to distinguish your suit as a cut above the mass-market offerings are:

- Working cuff buttons (to enable the loosening and folding up of sleeves for work and the washing of hands).
- Special silk linings.
- Monogramming and personalisation.
- The wearing of braces with trousers instead of a belt.
- Pairing a jacket with a waistcoat.
- The addition of accessories such as a buttonhole, lapel pin (military insignias are ideal), or pocket square.
- Elevating your suit with a custom made overcoat, a walking umbrella and a hat to match.

Button Etiquette: Note that with regards to the buttoning of a single breasted jacket, the top button (top one or two on a three buttoned suit) should be buttoned when standing. All buttons undone when sitting. The bottom button *never* buttoned. For double breasted jackets, the rules are a little more relaxed for every day business wear. All buttons can be closed when standing, or the bottom button remaining undone, neither look is a faux pas. Open buttons on a double breast if you wish when sitting, the extra fabric may look sloppy, but how comfortable you feel about this is personal preference. If you wish to flatter the military styling of the suit then keep buttons closed when sitting *and* standing. If attending a formal event in a double-breasted jacket, keep *all* buttons closed when standing and sitting.

Suppliers: Cordings of Picadilly, Gieves & Hawkes, Huntsman, Benson & Clegg, Turnbull & Asser.

Shirting

Shirts are the backbone of a gentleman's wardrobe. Appropriate in almost any setting, one must have a good selection to see him through most events in the year. Disregard pattern as what makes a shirt refined, and instead concentrate on the cut and fabric. The type to buy is the one most flattering to your body shape. A lean man may appear drowned in a classic fit, while the larger gent as though he is about to explode from a slim and highly tailored shirt. It pays to visit a *specialised* shirt retailer or ideally a tailor who will fit you for collar length and advise you on the best fit for your body shape and comfort requirements. The type you buy depends on your lifestyle, but the following styles are most versatile.

The **Oxford Cloth Button Down**, or OCBD, is a building block of the gentleman's wardrobe. It has remained at the top of the heap for over 120 years due to its versatility, popularity and ability to help the wearer look pulled together in almost every scenario. Whether worn for work or play, it is truly one of the most timeless pieces to obtain. Softer in construction than a classic dress shirt, the OCBD is made exclusively from a thick woven fabric called Oxford cloth, featuring a distinctive textured weave making it incredibly hard-wearing. With a classic fit, barrel cuffs, and a medium width collar (often buttoned down), this shirt can be dressed up or down depending on mood.

The **Dress Shirt** is made from superior grades of cottons and designed to be worn with your smartest suit for work, weddings, funerals, and formal events. Found in plain and fancy (herringbone and waffle) weaves, the man starting out should opt for basics of white to first populate his wardrobe and build from there. Medium spread collars and button cuffs will see you through most events, but if you are a fan of cufflinks then double cuffs look very smart. Shirt pockets on the dress shirt are for show only, and are never intended for use. Many shirt-makers offer a variety of colours, patterns and prints for the fashionable and trend setters, but for a classic English wardrobe stick to solid, restrained colours which complement your suits. Blues are a classic choice, and if flattering to your skin tone, consider pastels.

When an Englishman wishes to play with casual style he turns to **Tattersall & Country Shirts**. Classic, restrained and still fun (in the British sense), Tattersall and Country flannels or brushed cottons are paired beautifully with casual trousers, tweed blazers, novelty ties, waistcoats, and the country fleece or quilted gilet. Tattersall shirts consist of a large or small gridded pattern in two or more complementary colours making them very easy to pair with different items in the wardrobe. They were originally inspired by the blankets worn by thoroughbreds at Newmarket. As you can imagine, being so synonymous with country and equestrian wear, the colours making up the checks are often muted in natural shades on a cream or neutral background, but more adventurous colours such as purples and bright neons can now be found. Stick with earth tones for a gentrified look.

Linen Shirts feel beautifully soft and cool when worn, and are best coupled with weekend attire such as jeans, chinos, and shorts for effortless summer style. Wear with upturned or rolled sleeves for casual nonchalance, tucked or untucked.

The **Short Sleeved Shirt** is available on the high street, but not generally worn by the gentleman, or regularly found in the stock of his regular retailers. If he wishes to don short sleeves due to hot weather, he either rolls his casual shirts up at the lower sleeve and loosens a top button or two. Or he opts for a classic **Pique Polo** shirt instead which offers a smart yet more casual offering over a tailored shirt. Pair with jeans, chinos, or summer shorts.

Particulars on shirt detailing:

Pockets. Formal attire requires a shirt *without* pockets on the breast. While one is acceptable for informal wear, two pockets on the breast is for casual wear only. Shirt pockets are not usually intended for use. If you do, avoid popping any leaking pens in the pocket, lest you find yourself with a cliché ink stain.

Darts, Vents & Pleats. Designed to give ease to the shirt or pull the silhouette in, the less darting and additional seams across the torso of the shirt, the looser the fit will be. Pleats are often seen on the back yoke of a classic fit shirt, allowing for greater ease of movement across the shoulders and back. Pleats are a better option for the broader or heavier set gentleman with darts providing a trimmer silhouette, and looking best on formal and work wear shirting for the slim.

Collars. Smart and formal occasions call for as plain a design in the collar as possible. The 'button down' collar is seen as informal. After it was noted that English polo players were pinning their collars down to stop them from flapping up during a game, a collar that could be buttoned to the shirt was designed providing a less formal, more sporting vibe than a traditional point collar. Collar styles, widths and lengths vary greatly and your choice will depend on your personal preference. Steer clear of avant-garde pointed collars or anything too fussy if you wish to retain a classic look.

Cuffs. The most informal style of cuff is the button or barrel cuff, closed by a singular button. They are most seen on informal shirting—wear these shirts with casual sports blazers, tweeds and when adding a pullover to your look. Double cuffs, or French cuffs as they are also known, are double the length of a regular cuff and folded back on itself, are designed to be worn with cufflinks or fabric knots and offer a formal look. These look particularly smart when peeking out of the sleeve of a sharply cut suit.

Suppliers: Alan Paine, Cordings of Picadilly, Charles Tyrwhitt, Emma Willis, Gant, Hackett, Hawes & Curtis, T.M. Lewin, Musto, Purdey.

Knitwear

Modern knitwear offers an array of options in man-made fabrics and styles, but the gentleman will do best to keep to natural fibres and classic styles if he wishes to keep warm, as opposed to fashionable in our frigid British temperatures. It must be noted that garment care instructions for authentic knitwear requires a commitment to hand washing and delicate care-taking. However, should you devote yourself, nothing will compare for style or warmth. Heritage knitwear can thankfully still be sourced and the age of the internet has made heritage, geographically synonymous styles available to us all. Natural-fibre knits offer the man a superior way to keep the chill at bay while retaining a quality, classic look. Above this, one should feel proud to promote traditional craftsmanship and the support it provides to artisan producers in the UK.

The **Aran Sweater** takes its name from the Aran Islands off the west coast of Ireland, it's an iconic, instantly recognisable garment connecting people all over the world to Irish heritage, through generational ties or sheer fondness. Traditionally, garments knitted in Aran were made from cream coloured undyed and unwashed wool that retained its natural lanolin, making the final product water-repellent. Modern production is now mostly made up of washed 100% wools, or merinos and cashmere, styled into pullovers, vests, cardigans, half-zip sweaters, and accessories. The classic cable design long sleeved, crew-neck pullover is most traditional. Hand knit options are available, though pricier than a machine knit garment. The history of the Aran jumper is shrouded in mystery, some saying the technique is ancient, while others offering facts to the contrary, making the garment birthed as recently as the late 1800s by enterprising fisherman's wives who knit them for their husbands and to sell for additional household income. Regardless of the historical uncertainty, the Aran style of knit is traditional, hard-working and perfect for pairing over a Tattersall or country shirt for winter warmth.

Suppliers: Blarney Woollen Mills, Peregrine, James Meade.

Another traditional sweater with local heritage connections is the **Guernsey** or *Gansey*. Knit by the wives of seamen on the Channel Island of Guernsey to supplement household income since the eighteenth century, Guernseys were adopted for use by the British Royal Navy in the nineteenth century (and said to be worn at the Battle of Trafalgar). Traditional styling features include no discernible front or back, rib knit cuffs and neckband, and is tightly knit in 100% pure British wool to keep out the wind. As a hard working garment, each sweater is constructed 'in the round', meaning it has no seams. The gussets under the arm and at the neck, as well as the splits at the hem offer ultimate ease of movement. A variety of colours are available including red, bottle green, stripes, and neutrals. Some historical patterns which evolved from plain beginnings romanticise sailing; a rib at the top of the sleeve depicting a ship's rigging, the raised seam across the shoulder a rope, and the garter stitch panel is said to represent waves breaking upon a beach. Four hundred years later the practical design is still going strong. A choice in navy is most traditional and looks smart worn for sailing and country weekend pursuits over checkered shirts or thrown on over an undershirt. Pair with jeans or chinos and deck shoes for finer weather. With wellingtons or walking boots and under a waxed jacket in wetter weather.

Suppliers: Guernsey Woollens.

Fair Isle or Norwegians are handsome but rugged sweaters that offer a stylish and colourful alternative to keep out the chill. Traditional styles offer no more than two or three complementary colours. Avoid obvious motifs such as snowflakes if you wish to extend seasonal wearability.

Suppliers: Dale of Norway, Edinburgh Woollen Mill, Orvis, Peter Christian.

The wearing of **Cardigans** are a look not many can pull off. Favoured as a layering option by the teaching and lecturing professions, a gentleman with quiet confidence can wear one with his favourite tweeds, or casual shirting and moleskin, or needlecord trousers. Best reserved to potter about at home, there is not much else that screams 'English country gent' than a cable knit button up cardigan.

Suppliers: The House of Bruar, Peter Christian, Edinburgh Woollen Mill, John Smedley, James Meade.

Fine spun and lightweight **Crew or V-neck Sweaters**, pullovers, slipovers and vests in lambs wool, merino, and cashmere are staple layering for the man about town or country. Wear over shirts and ties or base layer t-shirts for additional warmth. Good quality and reasonably priced models are available from traditional menswear retailers offering you the chance to stock up on a variety of styles and co-ordinating colours for the shirts you wish to wear under them. Care must be taken with finer knitwear to keep them from pulls, pilling, or falling out of shape due to neglectful laundering.

Suppliers: *James Meade, Cordings of Picadilly, Hackett London.*

Polo, Roll, or Turtle Neck Sweaters are dashing when worn under a smart blazer or flying jacket for a smart off-duty look, and give off great James Bond vibes. If the knit and material is fine gauge then it is best left to the fit and trim as they expose every flaw. The heavier gentleman can wear thicker knits and cables. Wear over an undershirt making sure they themselves are lightweight enough so that the seams do not show through. This style of sweater is a great way to give a smart suit a casual air.

Suppliers: *Gant, Orvis, Ralph Lauren, John Smedley.*

Sport Jerseys or the **College Rugby Top** is the ultimate sweater for off-duty wear. Favoured as a coupling to jeans, sports trainers, boots, or wellingtons, the Rugby or Jersey is an ideal companion on weekends. Offering a nod to your favourite sporting team, for maximum authenticity source yours from your alma mater or local rugby team's official kit shop.

Suppliers: *Ryder & Amies, Crew Clothing, Hackett London, or official college and sporting stores.*

Fleece & Sweatshirts are your 'common or garden' way of staving off the chill. There is not so much of a 'traditional air' about them but they serve you very well in English winters. Source fleece from specialist outdoors and country-wear outfitters. Sweatshirts are often a fine way for a company to not so subtly advertise their brand on the chests of hipsters and the like. If you don't mind this then go ahead, but an Englishman wouldn't be seen dead emblazoned in a beer brand's logo or sports team insignia. Keep logos as small as possible for maximum style.

Suppliers: *For practical and subtle brands; Schöffel, Patagonia, Musto.*

Tennis or Cricket Jumpers are as classic as they come. Featuring a deep v-neck in a deeply ribbed or cable knit weave with long sleeves, or sleeveless, the Cricket jumper is synonymous with traditional English sporting style. Always in a shade of white or cream wool with one or two bands (to match your college, sports team, or regiment colours) along the neckline, and sometimes wrist or waistband. Wear yours over a casual shirt and tie (ideally an OCBD in a neutral colour), or over a white polo top for a casual sporting air. Can be paired with jeans for a casual take on a traditional look.

Suppliers: Luke Eyres of Cambridge, Smart Turnout London, Rochford Sports.

Novelty Sweaters are wickedly entertaining at Christmas, and cheeky slogan knits being a particular favourite of the 11th Duke of Devonshire. Always wear yours with nonchalance without any expectation of being taken seriously. Occasional forays into silly knitwear is unexpected and cuts a quirky dash in an otherwise serious reputation, However, consistent wear does nothing but appear juvenile. Know your moments.

Trousers

One cannot be seen without one's trousers. Unless enjoying the very height of summer in a pair of shorts, or heaven forbid swim wear, a gentleman is resigned to covering his bottom with the humble trouser. For workwear his bottom half is usually bedecked in a fabric to match his suit, or at the very least in a suitable co-ordinating option. Younger generations seem hoodwinked into believing there is only a singular choice of trouser for casual wear, obviously being the jean—but far superior and stylish options are out there for the taking, helping to raise his sartorial presentation from pedestrian to posh.

Moleskin Trousers, similar to jeans in cut and construction are comfortable, durable and stylish. They make a perfect choice for smart-casual occasions or dress down Friday at work, which take you effortlessly straight to the pub. A perfect accompaniment to tweed blazers and country shirts, moleskin trousers or moleskin jeans come in a vast array of colours to co-ordinate with any look. Choose navy to dress down a workday dress shirt, while muted neutrals work well with merino knitwear, rugby jerseys, aran knits, and tattersall shirts. The brushed pile of the fabric makes them supremely soft, warm and smart, but still a pleasing and comfortable trouser of choice for casual days. Most are cut in a traditional style, wear with a belt, tuck in your shirt, pair with a pullover, your Derby shoes, Chelsea boots, or loafers for smart casual go-anywhere ease.

Wool or cotton twill **Slacks** are the kind of traditional trousers your dad, uncle, or grandfather wore on the weekend for all sorts of home and leisure pursuits, before jeans were considered acceptable or *cool* for anyone other than teenagers. These are the typical off-duty trouser you'll find if you research wartime casual fashion for men. Cut rather loose with permanent creases and a pleated front, they make a good choice for smart casual occasions when one doesn't want to wear a blazer but wishes to appear more dressed up than had he chosen a jean or chino. Of course they still can be dressed up with said blazer and tie, as well as down. Wear yours with an Oxford, Derby, or brogue shoe and pair with a casual shirt or fine gauge sweater and a sport or bomber jacket. Cotton polo shirts and loafers are permissible to wear with slacks that are lightweight in both fabric and colour for summer wear. Winter options are wool, tweed, or a 'cavalry twill' favoured for its durable quality and extra warmth.

Chinos are the ultimate off-duty trouser, ready to pair with almost anything in the wardrobe and a godsend to wash. They are superior to jeans in the smart look they offer, as well as the wide range of colour options from sand, olive, and mustard through to the country gentleman's favourite staple 'tomato'. Cut like a jean they come flat-front or pleated, and in varying weights of fabric for year-round suitability. Opt for pleat front chinos for smart wear and pair with Derby shoes or desert boots. Plump for flat front slimmer styles which can be turned up at the ankle if desired for wearing in the summer with loafers or deck shoes. Keep your colours season appropriate and leather belts complementary to the environment in which you wear them. Braided, needlepoint, embroidered and 'polo' style belts pair best with lighter fabrics and colours, plain dark leather buckle belts with conservative and muted shades.

Corduroy Trousers are made of an incredibly warm and durable fabric, which is in essence a ridged style of velvet. Available in a finer needlecord or more often 'jumbo', the number of the 'wale' indicates the thickness of the ridges, the lower the number the wider the wale; for instance an '8 wale' is seen in most corduroy trouser production. Reserved for country wear, entry level colours to play with are evergreen, burgundy, and mustard—though corduroys aren't really corduroys unless they shout from the rooftops in the most outrageous colours. It's half the fun of wearing them. They look fabulous with a tattersall shirt and tweed or wool blazer sporting leather elbow patches. Sometimes clashing your trouser colour to the rest of the outfit presents a 'couldn't care less, *Lord of the Manor*' look. Corduroys must ideally not be paired with anything other than a lace up brown or tan brogue. At a push, tucked into wellingtons is acceptable. Most corduroy trousers look out of place unless one has a spaniel firmly at heel.

Denim Jeans, though not classically English (in fact, rather 'all American') have become so cemented to our sartorial identity that we have begun to think they are appropriate for all occasions, they are not. These trousers were intended to be a tough and rugged workhorse suitable to clad the bodies of the hard-labouring man. Prospectors, miners, farmers and cowboys wore them to *work*, and work hard they did. It can't be said a man working in an office will find he requires such a heavy twill to perform his duties. If you must opt for jeans for *weekend* wear, then shop for yours from some of the oldest jean brands in the world: Levi, Wrangler, or Lee. Buying designs as old and tried and tested as theirs will ensure a classic cut and durability, exactly as was intended in the original manufacture over a hundred years ago. A gentleman will steer clear of 'fashionable' jean cuts and colours and will opt for traditional 'blue jeans' in classic straight legged style such as the Levi 501 Original Fit.

Linen Trousers come in light or heavyweight fabrics. The thickness you require depends on the dress code of the event and the company to be kept. Summer holidays abroad with family and close friends make lighter weight linens appropriate, but summer soirées in the Isles in the presence of lords and ladies call for a tailored heavy linen. Still lighter than a regular trouser, tailored linen looks fabulous with a matching jacket and half basket-weave Derby shoes for a garden party, casual outdoor weddings, watching the cricket, or cheering on your chosen boat on the Thames. The general rule of thumb is 'if there are to be marquees, then linen is permissible'. Don't forget to don your white cotton or straw woven Panama.

Shorts are the reserve of the gentleman *abroad*. Rarely, unless he is sailing or camping in the British Isles will a gentleman require the use of shorts. In either case a pair of heavy cotton twill, 'utility' or chino shorts will serve him well. When on holiday a gentleman must refrain from thinking his polyester swim wear is an acceptable substitute for shorts for anywhere other than on the beach or relaxing poolside. When venturing into town or to dine, chino, tailored cotton, or linen shorts are cool, stylish and above all appropriate. The length of his short must ideally hit just above the knee and never be shorter than mid-thigh. Past sundown it is best to opt for linen trousers. Pair shorts with Birkenstocks, sandals, or boat shoes.

Suppliers: Crew Clothing, Cordings of Picadilly, Gant, The House of Bruar, James Meade, Peter Christian, Orvis, Oliver Brown.

Accessories

Accessories for the man are optional and entirely dependent on his personal tastes, and whether he wishes to decorate elements of his style. While there are items which are surplus to requirement, there are a few accessories that would be of benefit to have on hand.

Neckties have a reputation for being uncomfortable, but they are to a gentleman the same as a pair of heels to the woman. Insufferable perhaps, but ultimately smart and appreciated by the opposite sex when worn like you mean business. Neckties express your level of effort, accountability, and investment into the task or social occasion at hand. At the very minimum every gentleman should have two ties, one for smart occasions, church, and office wear (if he doesn't work in an office, something in which to meet a solicitor or his offspring's headmaster is still of use), as well as a country tie, in order to smarten up a tattersall and elevate his look. Ties are always subject to personal taste and artful ones are a delightful way to express oneself. The options are limitless, as is the expense for some of the finest ties.

Concern yourself first with collecting a variety in different colours to match shirts and suits before novelty options and wacky prints are considered. Weaves, herringbones and small prints make a simple solid colour look interesting. Fun, floral and flamboyant ties are suited to the gentleman who is confident enough to pull them off but considered inappropriate for serious work—save them for evening. Plain, geometric and small even prints are best for the office. The rural themed tie featuring labradors, pheasants, and shotguns are better suited for staying right there in the country. If one wishes to restrain himself entirely from the tie and such flamboyances, at the very least his regimental stripes, a simple dark navy basketweave or paisley silk for town and a wool/ tweed mulberry or evergreen for country use will serve him well.

Depending on the trend of the moment, the necktie can be narrow or wide, the gentleman who opts for a classic look should stick to a wider tie to avoid looking like a dandy. The Prince Albert, four-in-hand, half Windsor and Windsor knots are most conservative, with step by step instructions on how to achieve these knots widely available online. The bottom point of your tie should reach the middle point of your belt or waistband, and there should be no gap between the top of knot and your buttoned collar. Refrain from just loosening your necktie when hot, instead remove it entirely and undo your top shirt button (no more)—the 'half-removed' look is indecisive and messy.

The **Bow Tie or 'Dickie'** isn't reserved solely for black tie events. Those that fancy a quirkier 'Old University' look, particularly if working in teaching or lecturing professions, can pair a bow-tie in a casual fabric (not silk) with shirts and knitted pullovers for a smart striking effect without appearing too stuffy. The dickie-bow when worn in the daytime adds an element of fun to an otherwise staid outfit. Those of a snobbish persuasion would insist you choose a traditional dickie which you self-tie. Concern yourself with that if it bothers you, otherwise purchase ready-tied which always look perfect, and save yourself time and frustration. Options can be found at most smart outfitters in solid silks, wools, knits, and prints.

Scarves for gentlemen fall into two camps. Those to be worn to stave off the cold, and those to be worn for fashionable effect. Narrow and sometime tasseled **Evening Scarves**, draped around the neck or over the shoulders are an elegant addition to a white or black tie ensemble in winter. To stand out from the crowd at such an event is ungentlemanly and rather caddish, so choose yours in 100% silk *plain* black, ivory, or white. The more adventurous and outrageous man will choose flamboyant prints and saturated colours. **Dress Scarves**, appropriate for the commute to work are the kind you find in finer woven fabrics such as cotton or pashmina. Usually printed in paisleys, checks, and patterns they look smart paired with tailored overcoats. Choose refined colours of navy, camel and burgundy for your first foray. Remember, when the coat is removed, so is the scarf. **Casual Winter Scarves** in lambswool, fleece, or cashmere, or knitted wool in your old school colours, or an **Aviator Scarf** are best for off-duty and weekend wear. To continue to wear a winter scarf with anything less than a coat can look foolish and try-hard—remove the jacket, remove the scarf.

The **Pocket Square** is the hallmark of a gentleman who knows how to dress elegantly and looks very fine with his smartest suits. In order to achieve a harmonious look it is best to choose your pocket square in a shade and fabric flattering or complementary, but not matching, the necktie lest you look like a lost groom. Do not wear a pocket square if you are omitting a tie. There are various methods and ways in which to fold a pocket square which can be researched online, but the general rule of thumb if one wishes to save himself from such trivialities is to stuff it loosely inside of itself in the pocket and so that no outer edge or pointed corner is visible or sticking out. Aim for a 'cloud like' effect with beautiful ripples and peaks of fabric just visible in the pocket opening. Remember, the pocket square serves no purpose other than to elevate your outfit, one does not blow his nose into it or use it to mop his brow. Beautiful hand rolled silks, cottons, and linens are available. Store folded and launder with care.

Suppliers: Charles Tyrwhitt, T.M. Lewin, Hawes & Curtis, Huntsman, Eton Shirts, Savile Row Company.

Belts & Braces are without question necessary for the gentleman who wishes to keep his trousers where they belong. How much variety to have in one's wardrobe is the reserve of the individual, but at the very least a plain buckle leather belt in black, dark brown, and tan to match his shoes, and a casual needlepoint or woven leather belt for weekend wear is advised. Braces, whether elastic or fixed with clips or button loops can be worn with anything from a three-piece suit to country corduroys, and is a classic look somewhat rare in modern times. Braces featuring metal clasps are versatile to wear with many smart trousers (never jeans, linen or chinos), but traditional styles requiring permanently fixed brace-buttons are generally only found on pieces offered from a bespoke or high-quality tailor.

Suppliers: *Crew Clothing, The British Belt Company, Farrar Tanner, Pampeano, Tim Hardy, British Braces.*

Gloves should be of a slim-fit leather (or a vegan equivalent) if you are wearing them for business or commuting to work. Cashmere, silk, and fur-lined options are available for an extra barrier against the cold. Suede gloves with a fleece lining or merino wool are suitable for casual weekend wear. Driving gloves make a fun choice for motoring enthusiasts but should not be paired with suits. White evening gloves in unlined kidskin or Nappa leather (sometimes found in cotton or silk) are for white tie events and should one wish, the opera or theatre to pair with dinner jackets or top hat and tails. Remove gloves and place in the lap or a pocket when eating or drinking.

Suppliers: *Aspinal of London, Dents, Gant, Hackett, Pickett London.*

Cufflinks are beautiful accessories for the man, being so small and inconspicuous they are a fabulous way to add a touch of luxury to an outfit without seeming flamboyant. A ready supply of cufflinks in a variety of shades of silk knot, and plain gold or silver to complement the skin-tone is advised at first, oval shaped discs being a classic. Work from there expanding your collection and options with engraving, enamel, novelty shapes and gem-set. Take care with silver cufflinks as any tarnishing can rub off on fabrics making your cuffs appear shadowed and dirty. Periodically clean, buff, and shine all cufflinks, they are high traffic so can easily pick up dirt and debris.

Tie-bars, Clips & Pins are another way for a gentleman to show off his good taste. Aside from aesthetic value, the tie bar is useful to the working man for keeping his tie neat and protected from blustery wind, dropping onto his desk, into his lunch, or from dangerous equipment. Use yours to affix your tie securely to the button placket of your shirt. The positioning and placement of a tie bar should be between the third and fourth button of your shirt, around the area of your sternum, always affix in a perfectly horizontal line. The length of a tie bar should never be wider than the tie, ideally reaching three quarters of the way across. Before closing the tie pin, lift the top layer of tie up by half a centimetre or so to add ease of movement and keep the pin from pulling the tie down from your neck. An ever so slight curve in the tie is visually appealing. Unless he favours flamboyant styles, tie bars should be kept as plain or subtly patterned as possible in gold or silver, ideally his metals should match. If one is wearing silver cufflinks, his tie bar should also be silver. If one is wearing a pullover or waistcoat a tie bar should *not* be worn. The purpose of the bar is to keep the tie in place, additional layers make a bar redundant.

Suppliers: Aspinal of London, Gant, The family jeweller.

With regard to **Jewellery**, the English gentleman would consider nothing more than an engraved gold signet ring for his little finger and/or a wedding band. Anything additional to this is unnecessary and smacks of boasting wealth and professing vanity. He saves the purchasing of (tasteful) jewellery to bedeck his wife and daughters.

The wearing of **Watches** is a matter of personal preference, as is how many one wishes to own. To the gentleman concerned with time-keeping (as he should be) then choosing a style and price point of watch to wear should be commensurate with his lifestyle, interest in timepieces, and budget. At the very least, a casual 'daily' watch featuring a simple, no-nonsense slimline round watch face and leather strap will match almost all outfits. A dress watch in gold or silver-tone can be selected for evening wear if he wishes. For social occasions it is generally considered impolite to wear a watch, this rule has relaxed in the last few decades but to observe proper etiquette, omit a watch when dining formally or visiting the theatre or opera. Please note that to express one's wealth with the wearing and peacocking of a wristwatch is considered rather gauche. They are there to help you with timekeeping, nothing else, and you are only able to wear one at a time.

Suppliers: Citizen, Longines, Rotary, Timex.

Briefcases, Bags & Wallets are indespensible accessories for the gentleman working in the city or commuting with paperwork in tow. A classic-framed briefcase (also known as an attaché) in black leather, or a softer constructed leather satchel or folio in a favourite colour will look smart. Any weekend bag or wallet should also be of leather or vegan alternative. A smart wallet will transcend all outfits and social situations, whereas a casual wallet will not. Make sure to regularly clean and treat the leather as often as your shoes for maximum lifespan.

Suppliers: Aspinal of London, Cambridge Leather Satchel Co, Maxwell Scott, Mulberry, Pickett London, Smythson.

With regards to pants (of the English variety), not much can be said about **Underwear** without sounding unsavoury, yet nevertheless there are rules of conduct which must be adhered to. Wear what feels most comfortable to you, be it a brief, boxer, or y-front. What you choose is of no concern to anyone else, nor should they try to advise you otherwise—what is trendy or sexy does not concern your undercarriage. Comfort, cleanliness, and coverage are key.

Change it daily and once a hole appears or elastic fails send that item packing on a one-way trip to the rubbish bin. Your trouser waistband should fit, so make sure never to expose the waistband of your underwear or anything which should be covered by it when bending or reaching. The idea of underwear is to cover and conceal, not to be seen. 100% cotton, quality, and plain conservative colours are your only consideration. **Undershirts or Vests** in plain white jersey cotton are comfortable and useful for cold weather and additional layering, but be mindful of wearing with thinner shirts where they may be visible, it will undermine any desire you had to look smart. Wear instead when pairing a shirt with a pullover so that they may not be seen through the weave of a single shirt layer. With **Socks**, the same rules apply. 100% cotton in conservative colours (fun, novelty socks are the reserve of weekends, if you must). Launder after every use (they have a 24 hour time limit), throw away and replace the moment a hole appears, the elastic fails, or the fabric wears thin at the heel. Extend the life of your socks with regular trims of your toenails and buffing of hard heels.

Suppliers: Marks & Spencer, John Lewis, The Sock Shop.

The responsibility and care taking of a wardrobe

The care of a gentleman's clothing and accessories, once the responsibility of his valet, is now very much the concern of the gentleman himself, or if she is willing and happy to do so, his adoring and wonderful wife. With most of us belonging to a "throw it in the washing machine and forget about it" culture, one who wishes to refine and collect a worthwhile collection of clothing must take it upon himself to have a greater concern for the longevity of his investment. Bespoke tailoring, heritage and natural fabrics and handmade items must be worn and stored with great care. Each item should come with its own care instructions, take note of them and follow to the letter. Aside from this, here is a list of items that will help to protect and nourish your investment as much as possible:

- **Shoe Trees.** Intended to keep the shape of your shoes. Available in plastic, but far nicer and planet friendly options are available in cedar wood which also help to deodorise. Optional engraved brass plaques an upgrade.
- **Valet Box.** Invest in a specialist kit which includes all polish, creams, brushes, and cloths to keep shoes and leather goods clean and nourished.
- **Shoe Bags.** Buy in brushed cotton to protect shoes and surrounding items during travel.
- **Cedar Blocks.** Rings, blocks, and hangers protect your natural fibre clothing from moths. Place in wardrobes and in drawers to prevent a feast.

- **Hat Boxes.** Stuff the crown of your hat with tissue paper and store in boxes to prevent damage.

- **Wooden & Flocked Hangers.** A matching inventory keeps wardrobes uniformly spaced, look nicer, and flocking prevents items from slipping off.

- **Suit Carrier.** Invest in a breathable suit carrier to protect clothing when traveling.

- **Professional Clothes Steamer.** Consider investing in an upright steamer, it will save you from many a bind when a suit or shirt is pulled from the wardrobe last minute and there is no time to dry clean or iron.

Suppliers: Cathcart Elliott, Christy's London, Herring Shoes, Joseph Cheaney & Sons, The Holding Company.

Personal hygiene and grooming for gentlemen

Never before has there been such a vast divide between the man who couldn't care less, and the man so vain he spends as much time in front of the mirror as his female companions. With fashion and celebrity trends for 'beards' now appears a bevvy of grooming parlours for men on our local high street. Where once stood a traditional barber shop offering a 'short back and sides', Mr Vain can now enter any hipster establishment for a steam, facial, beard trim, manicure, and an eyebrow wax, all while enjoying a craft beer or two. We are not here to say that personal grooming is not in alignment with the English lifestyle, but rather 'over-preening' is. There is a certain ruggedness that is attractive in an Englishman, and no amount of fake tan or waxing that his competitor indulges in can distract from the Englishman's naturally weathered and casual appeal.

Skin & Shaving. Unless he suffers from a skin condition diagnosed by his doctor, an Englishman needs *nothing* more than a daily shave or close trim, a hot shower with soap, moisturiser for his face, application of deodorant, and a spritz of aftershave or scent. Shaving is a ritual unto itself and for a clean-shaven face it is said that nothing beats a wet shave using the finest razors and creams. If a moustache is worn it must be neatly trimmed and not overlap the line to the top lip. Given that shaving and the grooming of facial hair is something one must commit to daily, it pays not only to rise a little earlier to save himself from a 'rush job', but one should indulge himself with quality traditional shaving equipment and accessories to get the job done as pleasantly as possible.

Suppliers: Edwin Jagger, Floris London, Taylor of Old Bond Street, Truefitt & Hill.

Scents. Likely to be pre-approved by his wife, but the man hoping to *catch* a wife or make a good impression in the office must not overpower his aura with a less than quality fragrance. Traditional and attractive fragrances can be researched online, but sales pitch aside, nothing will stand the test of approval more than the noses of the man himself and his closest friends. Rather than deferring to the latest trends and what's 'cool', an Englishman will seek out a signature scent, and likely one that is not available at his local supermarket. There are a handful of heritage English perfume houses who know how to select a unique scent to complement the man. Always buy samples to test the chemistry against your body and whether they work with your personal taste and lifestyle before investing in full bottles. Trial the scent for at least a week before committing. Standard name-brand mass manufacturers sometimes offer smaller vials, though you will have better luck purchasing sample bottles and fragrance libraries from heritage perfumers.

Suppliers: Atkinson's of London, Bronnley England, Dr. Harris & Co, Floris London, Joe Malone, Miller Harris, Molton Brown, Penhaligon's.

Hair. Keep it clean, and keep it trimmed. If you have been blessed with a full mane it can look attractive if worn slightly longer, but the moment any thin patches or bald spots appear you are resigned to wearing it in a short back and sides. Traditional English haircuts are neither adventurous or trendy, instead leaning upon a military standard, and never *overly* styled with visible product. Pomades, pastes, and a little wax will keep hair in place but still looking natural. Venture not into the delusion that combing it over will hide hair loss, nor that dying out the greys will keep you young. A little bit of 'salt and pepper' on a man is most attractive and should you combine natural colour with a neat haircut on top of a stylish ensemble then the charisma only multiplies. Keep hair in check with regular visits to the barbershop, and while you are there ask him to garden your eyebrows, sideburns, and any nostril or ear hair that may be creeping beyond the confines of its orifice.

Suppliers: G.B. Kent & Sons, Truefitt & Hill.

Nails. Like the hair, nails should be permanently clean and kept trimmed short. If your barbershop offers a manicure service and you are happy to pay then leave the job to them. Best your hands and nails are serviced regularly than sporadically. Should you wish to DIY then a good nail brush, clippers, a file, and a cream are indispensable tools. While a man's hands are often lauded if they appear hardworking, cracked, sore, and callused paws are rarely attractive. Dirt under the nails is never acceptable and while unavoidable when gardening or performing routine motor or house maintenance, they must be cleaned at the earliest opportunity for appearance and the sake of your hygiene. Strike the right balance with a good slathering of rich hand cream before bed several times a week.

Teeth. Apparently the English are known for having bad teeth. Whether this reputation is deserved or not, a little crookedness can be charming, but bad breath is not. Brush twice daily, visit your dentist at least annually and make friends with breath mints. Chewing gum is déclassé and bad for the health, it's essentially akin to chewing on plastic. It looks and sounds disgusting, stay away.

Final notes on the English gentleman's style

Style is always a matter of personal preference, and with such a variety of clothing now considered 'acceptable' wherever you go, please be aware that whatever you clad yourself in will *always* be subject to scrutiny and opinions, welcome or not. The chapters above are an analysis of the English gentleman who wishes to be appropriate, conform to etiquette practices, and create a timeless appearance not a fashionable one. Do with the information what you will, but should you heed it to its full you may just find yourself experiencing a level of respect usually only reserved for the people who *look* like they deserve it. It's a funny *old* culture this English one, might as well embrace it and use it to your advantage, no?

An English Lady's Wardrobe

The classic Englishwoman also throws away any idea of wishing to be *fashionable* and instead turns her attention towards arranging for herself a wardrobe of beautifully tailored, timeless, and classic pieces that serve *her* for all occasions. So with this in mind, we will take upon ourselves the style anatomy of the 'English rose', a classic, demure, unassuming, and accessible style which is the perfect complement to the English gentleman.

A timeless and wholly 'unfashionable' wardrobe for ladies

It is a little sad that there is so much choice and inconsistency in women's fashion today. Unlike menswear, whereby we can clearly define the style of the gentleman, what constitutes classic style for the female isn't as black and white. The wide expanse of womenswear available in the modern age isn't necessarily a good thing. The amount of self-taught or academy trained 'stylists' ready and willing to help you weed through your wardrobes, tell you which colours suit your complexion, and willing to go shopping on your behalf, only demonstrates the level of confusion the fairer sex really suffer when it comes to fashion. Many who call upon a stylist do so out of frustration, feeling overwhelmed with choice and that their sartorial needs aren't met.

Such irritation can easily be rectified by adopting a few boundaries. This is achieved by raising the standards in the way you shop and dress. More importantly, listening to your *heart* regarding what you'd like to wear, not what the dear old editor of Vogue, Anna Wintour tells you.

One of the joys of becoming a woman, rather than spending life as an eternal girl, is that one can start to enjoy wearing what actually suits her lifestyle and makes one feel *comfortable* rather than pandering to the opinions of the latest fashion magazines. The greater pleasure of the English lady, is that she can treat her wardrobe like a fine art gallery and collect not only what will suit her, but what will last, perhaps for decades, and often will become heirlooms for her daughter. With the rise of fast fashion and the over consumption of cheap materials, never has there been a better time to go against the grain and make choices that are not only stylish but economically viable in the long run. Where there used to be four seasons of fashion, we are now seeing not only twelve, but sometimes fifty-two rotations of the rails on our high streets. It's impossible for mere mortals to keep with that pace darling, so do stop trying.

You already *know* whether you feel more comfortable in a pair of trousers or a skirt, or that a crew neck makes your bust look big. Frills may make you feel silly, but look charming on your petite little sister. Beige drains you and magenta makes you come alive. No one knows you more than yourself, so learn to place trust in that and that alone.

When the fashion magazines tell you that magenta is *out*, and that top-to-toe beige is trending for autumn/winter. What will you do?

This confusing and faddish global attitude to what a woman *should* be wearing breeds a feeling of discontent with one's wardrobe, as it is always apparently out of favour with the current trend, despite the fact that you made your purchase but a week ago.

Larkin's, ladettes and little dreams

"What is my style?" When we aren't crystal clear on the answer, this seemingly unanswerable internal debate leaves us with wardrobes bursting at the seams, yet we always feel we have nothing to wear. The true answer, surprisingly, cannot be found in the latest fashion magazine, but instead, I believe, lies in our past. In our childhood fantasies, memories, and expectations.

Q: As a girl, what did you dream of wearing when you grew up? What type of life did you think you'd have, and which ladies did you look up to?

You may need to think about this a little bit. Perhaps ponder over it for a few days and recall memories from your coming of age years.

For me, coming of age in the time of a midriff-bearing Britney Spears, I went along with the motions, but in my heart I ached for whimsical floral print midi-length Laura Ashley. I adored movies and books with a rural England, American pioneer, or farming and vintage theme; Charlotte's Web, Little House on the Prairie, Anne of Green Gables, Black Beauty, The Secret Garden being favourites. I spent my days at the feet of my grandparents in the flower garden and vegetable patches, chasing butterflies, or knee deep in ponds catching frogs. Camping in the woods down in Dorset featured heavily in my life, as did adventuring with a friend on weekends in the local heathland. On cold damp days indoors I played 'house', read voraciously, or watched and learned as hearty meals were cooked, or beautiful quilts were pieced together. I can still describe in much detail the outfits worn by Mariette Larkin portrayed by Catherine Zeta Jones in all episodes of The Darling Buds of May. From her floral dresses to her daily overalls. Special mention to the female cast of Little House on the Prairie, Seven Brides for Seven Brothers, and the Disney girls *before* their princess makeovers. In particular Aurora, barefoot in the forest, and Belle before she meets the Beast. Their simple provincial dresses, aprons, and cloaks stole my heart. They both carry a basket and Belle is always carrying or reading a book—my two favourite accessories, both of which I have in abundance. In my mind, Belle especially was a true heroine because of her gentle yet determined spiritedness. She traded her freedom to rescue her father and saved the day by winning over the hardest of hearts. Teaching by *example* how to be kind. Her simple quiet beauty and kindheartedness shone brightly, more so to me than her later ball-gown glamour.

It's clear to see I have a thing for simple but whimsical, feminine and girlish silhouettes in soft florals or spring colours, ribboned but 'undone' hair, floaty skirts, overalls or cotton dresses paired with wellingtons and cardigans. I like things that flatter the shape of a lady, but are still modest. Clothes that are pretty but in which you aren't afraid to get a little messy. I'm drawn to styles and prints that evoke a sense of practical homeliness, rural country life, femininity, springtime, picnics, and flowers. This is all worlds away from late 90s ripped denim, parachute trousers, and stomach flashing crop tops. Feeling like I had to wear all those things to fit in was devastating. It made me feel like a fish out of water, a black sheep, as well as the ugly duckling. I couldn't put my finger on it at the time though. I felt I had no *choice*.

Think about that for a minute, my fantasies not only demonstrated my personal style and tastes but my *values* and my dreams. I knew them even then. Even though the current trends shrouded them and I was too immature to recognise it. I wanted to be slightly vintage, to be ultimately feminine but still practical with it, and celebrate that part of me—not cool, not sexy, not hip and definitely not pop-current. What I wore to 'fit in' dulled my spirit. I was a light hidden under a bushel. The real me was hidden away according to the pattern of the world. What kind of life could I have had in those years if only I was unafraid to truly be myself?

Many of us still feel this way if we aren't living according to the desires of our heart. When you get swept up in the world, the high street, fashion magazines, and style 'gurus' ultimately make style decisions for you.

One of the most liberating things you can do is to *embrace* your inner eight year old. She had dreams and was prepared to chase them. Forward five years or so and we start listening to the world, which only makes us miserable. We are made unique, and so we should act accordingly. How does the uniform available on the high street help us achieve that? Are you happy with this status quo? Or are you frustrated that you aren't being true to yourself and what you like to wear? Teenage feelings of awkwardness can last for decades, even a lifetime, unless we still ourselves for a moment and take stock. Who are you dressing for and why? What in? **As grown women who have a choice, shouldn't we wear what makes us feel** *good*? Are we still not that child? We may be a little longer in the tooth perhaps, but our spirit is just the same. Sure we may have grown out of certain things here and there, but the very essence of what makes you 'you' likely hasn't.

Do I always dress like Mariette Larkin? No, but I know that **I feel at my best when I do.** As much as I can shoehorn those colours and prints into my day, there are times when only a practical pair of jeans, a t-shirt, or a big old puffer coat to keep out the cold would be appropriate. I'm aware enough of what's going on around me to choose my moments. We have to live with a connection to reality, but you can bet your last penny on the fact that as soon as an opportunity arises, out come those twirly skirts, florals and vintage Laura Ashley frocks. Being true to your personal style is keeping those stolen moments in mind, always. Never questioning what is in fashion *right now*, but asking instead *what do I want to purchase* out of the sea of 'options' that will have *me* excited to pull it out of the closet in five or ten years from now? Everyone needs *basics*, but what clothes really make you happy?

Today you might label my style as wholesome, practical, or a little 'librarian' in aesthetic. It takes some *doing* and deep thinking to finally arrive at a place that makes you feel so very comfortable and decisive about what you want to wear and what makes *you* feel good.

Maybe you think my girlish dreams typical for an eight year old and it's silly to reference them for curating style now I'm old, but are *your* interests much changed from when you were young? Did you love horses? Do you now lean towards country/equestrian wear? Maybe you were outdoors all the time, collecting bugs in overalls and running free. Do you like to hike and go camping still to this day? Perhaps you dreamed of city life and being a lawyer, sharp suits, minimalist silhouettes and tailoring are your thing. Did you want to run away and travel the world barefoot with nothing but a backpack? Is bohemian style and yoga appealing? Perhaps punk, or rock and roll set your world on fire and vintage band t-shirts are right up your street. Did you just want to rip off those bows and ribbons? Being made to wear a skirt or anything pink was the height of embarrassment and you wanted to get muddy like the boys. Today, jeans and a t-shirt or the 'Lagenlook' is oh so comfortable.

Maybe you *have* always adored the latest trends and are happy to shop until you drop and turn your style around on the beat of a wing. The important thing is to be *you*. With such variety in ladies fashion it is hard to see the wood for the trees. Much easier in menswear it has to be said.

What do you like? There is no wrong answer, every one of these preferences can be still be manipulated into helping you stay appropriate and look like a lady. This world would be too boring if we all looked the same, but equally it would still be nicer if everyone looked *presentable* and offered the best of themselves. Would that not make you feel happier in your skin and more embracing of others? Is it not easier to talk to and smile at a stranger who is nicely dressed and clean, than the sloppy Joanna who turned up at the supermarket still in her PJs…

Shallow judgment perhaps, but we naturally embrace what is comfortable and *makes us feel good*.

Happiness in the way you present yourself to the world will elevate every area of your life. People will smile at you, treat you better, and respect you— because you respect yourself! You don't have to dress exactly like a royal, an office worker, or be a carbon copy of the 'yummy mummy' in the playground in order to fit in or be considered well presented, but for the sake of your self-esteem and general etiquette there *are* social guidelines to follow. The same rules apply for the Larkin's *and* the ladettes.

Wait, what makes all this English or even related to etiquette?

Unlike our cousins in sunnier climes, we must clad ourselves in season-*appropriate* styles that can take us from the playground to the pub, or the city to the country pile. Where an English gentleman's wardrobe and what his tailors and outfitters supply is somewhat transferable from city to country and designed to last for decades. This is not the case for *most* of what's available for the lady. Male fashion hardly changes, whereas the cuts, fabrics, prints, and shapes of womenswear change so drastically from season to season, and quality is diminishing.

So we must find consistently stylish key pieces which will not only bring a lady joy when wearing them, but help her to dress appropriately and comfortably for all occasions. We must forget whimsical fads and instead dress for a mix of practicality and beauty, but practicality comes first, every time. The 'old-English' example, such as our matriarch the Queen, is rather restrained and fastidious when it comes to off-duty wardrobe. Things must be practical, serve a purpose, and not appear faddish. Wasting money on things that fly by night is the height of foolishness and doesn't wash with those who live a classic English lifestyle. Everything you purchase *must* have a way of serving you and provide real value for your lifestyle. Nothing is bought on a whim. If it isn't practical and of good quality it doesn't deserve a place in your life or your closet.

In essence, we are borrowing from the boys in terms of their *outlook and attitude* towards style and clothing. It must be of great quality and value, serve its purpose, feel comfortable, be versatile, and help one avoid having to return to the shops for as long as possible to replace it. Doesn't that sound liberating?

Here listed are styles, dressmakers, and designers for every clothing category that remains true to classic styling, hemlines, and standards of manufacture that will enable you to create a beautiful, anglo-approved wardrobe to see you appropriately through any event. We will also study the etiquette rules and ideals with regard to each *element* that makes up an English rose's wardrobe, as well as the considerations and the specifics to look out for when shopping for each category.

Raising standards, not hemlines

Natural, well made & timeless. The main rule of thumb when shopping for your new wardrobe is to invest in clothing and the accessories where applicable that are composed of 100% natural materials (or near enough). The expense of sourcing and purchasing good raw materials is a consideration to the manufacturer, so naturally standards of production will be higher, and this quality passes on to you. Consider also the timelessness and versatility of the garment and whether you are able, and willing to store and care for clothing correctly.

Less is more. We live in a 'more is more' culture, blinded by shiny and new things, but the lady will take no notice of this and turn her attention to the new adage 'best is best'. It is far better to invest in any item of your wardrobe that will withstand wear and washing far beyond what could ever be achieved from brands with less than ideal manufacturing practice and quality control. One great dress that will last for years is better than five that threaten to fade and fall apart within months.

Consider your current lifestyle above all else. If you are a country girl, is there really much need for tailored pieces and evening dresses in your wardrobe? Perhaps good quality denim and heritage knitwear that stand up to the elements is a better investment for you. Equally a lawyer in the city may have little need for chunky knitwear and flannel shirts if her weekends are spent doing yoga by day and out for dinner at fancy restaurants or the theatre at night. The changing tides of 'fashion' do not cater to differing lifestyles, just one section of society at a time, so you must blink and see the wood for the trees. What do you *do* with your time and how can your clothes best *serve* you? It's very lovely to shop for the life you *wish* you had, but far more practical and contented to dress appropriately for the one you have right now. Invest your money on practical things, rather than whimsy.

Demure and dignified, not flashy and fashionable. Regardless of her personal style, no matter what she chooses to wear, a lady knows that it is never appropriate to expose too much skin. Special attention is paid to necklines, hemlines, and the transparency of fabrics. Sexy doesn't have to mean exposed, and summertime is not an excuse to bare all.

Shop to replace. It's no use going into debt trying to obtain a quality wardrobe all at once. As things wear out, replace them only then. The environment already has so much strain on it that your fashion-fads will break the camels back if you throw them out before they've done their time. Consider whether you are able to source what you need secondhand. There are plenty of websites where you can find quality and gently used designer pieces at a fraction of the cost to buy it new. Get *over* your obsession with 'new' and help the planet a little. Even the smallest of ways makes a difference.

Secondhand doesn't mean second rate. I was bought a black Chanel classic-flap handbag (secondhand, made in 1993), by my husband as a treat when my first book 'Ladies Like Us' was published. It is in great condition, in fact barely used and was less costly than buying it new. I adore the fact that it's considered 'vintage' and has had a life before me. I hope that it will also have a life beyond me if I take care of it well enough. What's funny is that no one knows or has ever questioned whether it was purchased brand new. Oh and guess what, it's *still* a Chanel handbag! Just because some other lady took the hit on the depreciation doesn't make it any less lovely or valuable to me. When you really want to source something classic and potentially expensive for your wardrobe, consider vintage first. If you must have it *new* then evaluate your emotional ties to the experience. What will buying it new *give* to you? Is it worth parting with the extra cost for the exact same item? I also have a collection of vintage dresses and scarves, obviously purchased secondhand. Not only are they cheaper than buying new but I have never seen other ladies wearing them, a guarantee of sartorial individuality, if you will. It's also true that some things really do look better a little worn in, Levi's jeans are a perfect example.

Know the colours that suit you and remain faithful to them. Some women know by instinct what colours suit them, but for those that feel clueless it pays to have your colours analysed. It really does make shopping that bit easier and helps you to navigate the rails and only consider items from your colour wheel. Not only does it make shopping easier, but your entire wardrobe becomes harmonious in colours that look good on you, as well as complement each other. There are a number of expert companies offering this service. For a small fee and a few hours of your time, you come away with a little pocketbook of fabric swatches specific to your skin tone which prove an invaluable tool to take along on shopping trips and compare with clothes on offer.

Over time, not over credit limits. Rome wasn't built in a day, and neither was a classic wardrobe. Plan your shopping trip according to season and, if starting from scratch, what you need to replace *first* from your current wardrobe. It is no use saving for and investing in a designer silk summer dress in the depths of winter when you have a moth eaten coat and boots with holes in the soles. A lady shops smart and does not over-extend her budget because of a 'must have it now' mentality. Neither does she shop on impulse. A lady learns the art of delayed satisfaction. If she sees an item she likes, then she will try it on to see if it is suitable, then leave the store to think about it. Perhaps she may even sleep on it. If the item is still playing on her mind and she is certain it is of good quality, will complement her lifestyle and the rest of her clothing, only then will she return to the store to buy it. Yet not before researching whether it could be purchased at a discount online.

Go alone. The movies and popular women's shows have made out that shopping with your friends is meant to be fun, when in fact it is rather a foolish idea. Every woman is there for herself and, less than ideally, may give you false compliments in order to save face. Who wants to tell their friend that her bottom really does look fat? No two women have entirely the same taste, nor the same lifestyle, so a lady should rely on only herself to know what to purchase. Worse still is shopping with the enabler, who encourages you to buy one in every colour, or to purchase something on credit "because you deserve a treat, darling". Worse ever more is the shopping partner with a larger budget who makes you feel as though you have to keep up. Or the friend who makes you feel bad for 'spending so much' when she can hardly afford a new coat for winter. Learn to trust your own taste, instincts, and opinion. Despite a sorry lack of good publicity on the matter, husbands are surprisingly good shopping partners. They will be honest with you, both about what looks terrible and what they love to see you wearing. Just make sure not to wear them out with shopping for hours on end. Pick your moments and ask them to help with one or two key decisions.

Get help from the help. Learning to shop well and for quality items will likely bring you back to a few select retailers, so make friends with the managers and build rapport with the staff. The service when you return will be better than if you were just another face in the crowd. Not only that but the staff at quality fashion brands tend to stick around longer, know their products, have a keen eye for quality, and want to really help their customers—not just earn a wage. The standard of employment and job satisfaction for the staff is higher and makes it harder for Joanna-average to get a job there. The staff must have something 'about them' in order to win and keep their employment. Spend time in the store rather than rushing about and *tell them you are looking for xyz…* Let them do their job. If the style they present isn't right, or the quality isn't there, tell them so (kindly) and what you are willing to buy. "I really wanted something in a looser cut/warmer fabric/rounder neckline/higher waist/darker shade, etc". Over time your sales assistants will know what you like and become key players in helping to match pieces from current seasons with their older season items you purchased on previous visits. Trusted, quality brands have no business selling you the things you don't really need or like as you won't return. Quality is king, for both item and service.

Write a shopping list. As with grocery shopping, you should write a list of the things you require for your wardrobe. This not only helps to keep you mindful about *what* you purchase, but keeps you on budget and saves waste. Too many women are throwing away tonnes of unworn, unloved clothing in their lifetime. Enough is enough, if you care about the planet, helping to end child labour, and raising your personal standards, then raise the bar! We complain we have nothing to wear, but blindly enter cheap retail stores on a Saturday after pay day and grab at anything in our size and apparently 'on-trend', then swipe that plastic. Never really trying those items on first or considering whether said item is really *us*, whether it matches with any of our current items, or even how it makes us *feel*. Please consider whether you have an addiction to shopping (whatever end of the market you shop at) to fill a void in your life, and get some professional help if you do.

Seriously ladies, whenever you think or feel you need something new for your wardrobe, get a slimline notebook for your handbag, or create some notes on your phone about the item. Jot down the must-have features, where you'll wear it, and with what, then finally your ideal budget to put towards it.

Little Black Dress
- Plain. Crepe or suiting (matte black finish). Fully lined.
- Round or scoop neck. Straps wide enough to cover bra.
- Knee length.
- Pencil or A-line skirt.
- Work appropriate - wear with cardigans and blazer.
- Can be dressed up with heels and sparkle for dates or dining out.

- Will likely wear at least once a month - machine washable/able to iron?
- Budget £150 max.

When you have considered all these must-have details, you can begin to source the item. The internet is great for window shopping and perusing, but use it for just that initially. If you spot something you suspect aligns with your new shopping values, make time to visit the store if possible and try it on. Call ahead to see if they have one in stock and ask the staff to put it aside or order one in for you to try on. Given the level of quality you should be aiming for with regards to your clothing, the experience should be able to afford this kind of pre-thought, treatment, and consideration. Calling ahead to Primark and asking them to set aside a pair of trousers versus calling Hobbs to do the same will reveal to you just how much the brand care about their offering and how they sell it to you. Do you not deserve better? Of course, you may be spending five times as much, but a better quality item will last you five times as long, and look *more* than five times better. A deal isn't a deal when you have to keep repurchasing poor quality goods.

If you wish to purchase the item, ask the staff when the next sale is. If the answer is within the next couple of weeks, consider whether you are happy to take the risk and wait it out and see if you can get the item at a lower price. Otherwise, if the item hits all the right notes and you have the budget, then purchase the item, with gladness in your heart. Gladness that the item is exactly what you were looking for, makes you feel good when you put it on, and that you can *afford* it. Making these slow, considerate purchasing decisions not only builds a relationship between you and the item, the weight of the decision made helps you appreciate and value the item much more. Take the item home, display it on the front of your wardrobe for a day or two. Admire it and welcome it into your life! As William Morris said; *"Have nothing in your life that you do not believe to be beautiful, or useful"*. This extends to every item of clothing you wear, treat it all with respect and love. This may not be true of the things you have now, but make it a rule for the things you buy from now on. Every time you take that lovely piece out of your wardrobe you will remember the refined decisions you made in order to bring it into the narrative of your life. It will become part of your story and you will wear the clothes, not the other way around. *You* will dictate your style, not according to what is fashionable right now, which makes it all the more unique and beautiful.

Of course, anything you buy is merely a *thing*. We are told we shouldn't be concerned with *things*, but any clever sausage will know we all have to have some *things*. Isn't it far better that the things we have are the *best* things, not the *most* things.

A classic and appropriate lady's wardrobe

While your personal taste and what you feel comfortable wearing is completely up to you and should be considered according to your lifestyle, there *are* certain pieces that are considered to be the backbones of the wardrobe for any woman which will help her to be properly dressed according to occasion and season. The following is a list of clothing items, while not exhaustive, should be enough to flesh out the wardrobe to the point where a lady will *always* have something timeless and appropriate to wear no matter the dress code or event.

Dresses

The **Day Dress** is a staple for the lady. One should consider at first concentrating on buying simple dresses in patterns and colours that complement the British summertime, rather than trendy or tropical prints which only seem fitting when on holiday in far sunnier climes. When a dress sways more toward a classic style than current fashion, it lends itself to repeated wear over the years. Classic designs include the shift dress, shirt dress, wrap dress, tea-dress, and a-line tunic. Straps should be comfortable and thick enough to cover the bra and much of the shoulder, with necklines not extremely low as to expose too much of the bosom or cleavage. The skin in that area is prone to sun damage and an over-exposed hot and sweaty boob is not pretty. For these reasons, cover up.

Where shorter skirts may on the surface promise to be cooler, it is better to buy a knee length skirt in a looser fit for coolness and to keep you from too much sun exposure. Seats and surfaces absorb summer heat and to touch one with the back of a bare thigh is not comfortable. The ideal dress is loose enough to allow for breathing room between the skin and the fabric as well as catering for a little swelling which we all know happens to the best of us in the most extreme of heat waves. Materials should ideally be 100% cotton or linen and checked for sheerness. It is not ideal to have to wear a slip in such hot weather in order to protect modesty.

Summer Dresses can be worn for all casual occasions from picnics to summer garden parties, children's sports days to general daily errands, so the print and colour must be versatile enough to work across the board. Consider buying a few basic dresses in subtle shades that complement your skin tone. These can be dressed up or down with accessories before branching out into dresses with bolder prints. Basic designs and shapes such as the shift, a-line and tea dresses can be transferable from work to weekend, whereas ruffle details, beading, shirring, crazy overblown prints, tiered skirts, and the like are better suited to casual weekends and vacations. Pair your dresses with cardigans and light summer jackets, if they are a heavier fabric they may work well with a blazer. Depending on the length of the dress they can work well with a pashmina and light summer sandals then transition well into autumn when worn with knitwear, tights and boots—knee length dresses being the most seasonally transferable.

Jersey and Polyester Dresses are suited for casual wear, and work well for travelling when ironing may not be a priority or possible. With jersey dresses, make sure they are tailored to fit around the bust-line and just below it. Jersey tends to sag with its own weight over time, thus potentially leaving you exposed where you don't wish to be. Polyester can be incredibly light, but make sure to keep it loose in areas that may show or absorb perspiration, the material is not breathable. Skirt length is also a consideration with very lightweight fabrics, watch the wind doesn't catch your too-short skirt!

For a luxurious and semi-formal take on a day dress, consider silk. Silk looks particularly lovely when cut into a forties 'tea dress', the flow of the fabric offering unrivalled femininity and ladylike charm.

Basic day dress ideals:

- 100% cotton or linen that holds its shape.
- Material thick enough to negate the need for a slip.
- Block colours or small even prints.
- Simple design to dress up or down.
- Straps wide enough to cover the bra.
- Neckline and back not too low.
- Fit neither too loose or tight.
- Length no shorter than above the knee to protect modesty and from sun-exposure.

Suppliers: Hobbs, Seasalt, Mistral, White Stuff, Boden, Madeleine, Toast, Jigsaw, Joules, L.K. Bennett, Cath Kidston, Gant.

Consider learning how to **Sew Your Own Dresses**, or find someone who can do it for you. The ability to create a wardrobe of made to measure dresses in fabrics and shapes that you love (not what current trends dictate), is a lost art and pleasure most of us have never thought about. The ability to make your own dresses, blouses, and skirts was once a common skill held by ladies of all backgrounds. It is only since mass-manufacture and the ready-to-wear markets really kicked off that these once necessary and helpful skills have been lost. Sewing or knitting your own clothes may just be the liberating, productive, and worthwhile hobby you've been looking for.

The **Work Dress** intended for office environments is best purchased in solid colours with simple clean cuts in a knee length pencil shape. The neckline depends on your bust size; v-necks and scoops (not too deep) working for the larger bust, while slash necks and crew necks are better for ladies with a small bust. Ideally the dress should have sleeves, long, quarter length, or shorter, but at the very least sleeveless in design, which can be covered with a cardigan or jacket, but never 'strappy'. Colours are professional in black, navy, charcoal, deep maroons, greens, and blues. In summer, lighter colours can work but choose accessories with caution and keep them plain. Anything flowery or novelty can make it look as though you are off to an afternoon tea as opposed to a board meeting. When trying work dresses on, make sure to check how high the skirt rises on the thigh when you sit down, this may decide whether you require the wearing of tights to keep some level of modesty. Consider also the fit of the neckline and shoulders and whether they gape open when bending over.

Suiting fabrics, wools, and polyesters which keep their shape are ideal for the office, but heavier tailored jersey and scuba can work nicely in a semi-formal work environment.

The lady in the office needs to strike the right balance between professionalism and femininity. Don't be fooled into thinking that only a woman has to think about what she wears in order to get ahead at work. Both men and women need to be aware of keeping a conservative appearance in order to win respect, and a woman certainly won't win it by dressing exactly like her male counterparts. Embrace your curves, but keep your lines and cuts of dresses and suits feminine but demure. Necklines for the office should never show a hint of cleavage or expose roundness of your upper breast. Anything above the knee is inappropriate and shoulders should remain covered. These rules are there for the comfort of everyone—not for protection, not to make a point of anything, or anyone. If you wish to climb the corporate ladder based on your work talents, keep your physical talents under wraps and let that sexualised workplace narrative remain far from your professional experience.

Suppliers: Hobbs, L.K. Bennett, Whistles, Reiss, Jaeger, Winser London.

The **Little Black Dress**, commonly known as the LBD, is the dress in your arsenal for cocktails, parties, or award events. You might choose yours in another shade than black, such as red, or perhaps emerald, a navy, or another deep colour to suit your complexion. If you are to have but *one* evening dress make it as classic as possible in order for it to be as *versatile* as possible. Think of something Audrey Hepburn might have worn, it would have been pared back so much in style that the dress itself is barely noticeable, instead helping the woman to shine. You can alter your accessories to match the occasion, perhaps pairing the dress with a heavily beaded cardigan, cape, or a faux fur stole. Jewellery too can take your look from decent to decadent with a simple change from pearls to glittering diamonds (or lookalikes).

It is also possible to take this dress from conservative to 'can-can' ready with a switch from simple pumps to a strappy heel. They key is to let the accessories and how you style your hair and make up do the talking. While I don't usually promote the spending of astronomical amounts of money on clothing, since this is likely to be the *one* item that you shall return to again and again, it is warranted to pay for quality and really treat yourself on such a classic. If you choose and take good care, it could be something to pass on to a daughter. Ideally source a highly skilled dressmaker who can design and fit a dress for you perfectly, or save the money you would have spent on ten 'occasion' dresses from the high-street and purchase something from a classic high-end designer such as YSL, Alaïa, Roland Mouret, or Hervé Leger who really understand and design for this market. Websites such as Net-a-Porter or Farfetch make it a pleasure and easy to browse, far less intimidating and time consuming than shopping in boutiques, and they deliver to your door!

The anatomy of the perfect LBD:

- Sheath, pencil or a-line cut.
- Most fitted at the waistline.
- Skirt to the knee, just above, on, or just below.
- Concealed zip closure, no buttons, no exposed zips or tie detailing.
- Modest neckline in either v-neck, boat, or scoop neck to suit your shape.
- Simple wide straps, enough to cover the bra.
- Material in a semi-matte finish such as crepe, silk georgette, or cotton-gabardine.

Suppliers: *Hobbs, L.K. Bennett, Karen Millen, Coast, Goat, Beulah London, Reiss, Ghost, Phase Eight.*

Dreamy Designers: *Needle & Thread, YSL, Alaïa, Roland Mouret, Hervé Leger, Preen, Catherine Walker, Alexander McQueen.*

It would be remiss to refrain from mentioning suitable dresses for other occasions such as christenings, funerals, weddings, balls, black tie, and the like. However the guidelines of dressing for each event is somewhat similar, so we shall detail the etiquette and anatomy of the item according to occasion, not the particulars of the dress itself.

For a wedding:

• Do not wear white, or shades of cream. Shades of white are only acceptable if serving as a background to a dominant print in other colours.
• Skirts should not be shorter than the knee.
• Keep shoulders covered in churches or other places of worship.
• Fabrics should not be so thin or fine as to reveal undergarments, wear a slip if necessary.
• Avoid anything that threatens to expose more than you wish if you have one too many drinks. Steer clear of mini skirts and strappy dresses.
• The attention should be on the bride at all times, avoid avant-garde designs, inappropriate cutouts, and crazy embellishments on dresses and all accessories.

For a christening:

• The mood is happy, hopeful and a celebration of new life, dress in light, bright colours to suit the occasion.
• Modesty is key, children are present.
• Pair dresses with cardigans or light blazers and keep shoulders covered in places of worship.
• Fabrics and designs can be a little more casual than those worn for a wedding.
• Shoes should be conservative and not too high, there will be little children underfoot.
• A skirt, blouse and cardigan are also acceptable attire so long as they are modest.

For a funeral:

• You are paying respect, so dress respectfully.
• Knees and shoulders covered, nothing too tight.
• Shoes are modest, closed toe and heels low. You may be walking on uneven ground and grass if a burial is to take place.

- The family of the deceased may request that you wear bright colours as opposed to black. If you do not own a conservative dress in a solid bright colour, do not purchase a new outfit for the event, instead accessorise a basic darker toned shift or dark trousers (plus blouse) with bright pieces such as a cardigan, scarf, a bright bead necklace, or pashmina.

- A pencil skirt or smart trousers, blouse and cardigan or blazer is also acceptable attire so long as they are modest.

- Wear opaque or sheer tights depending on the season.

For a ball, black or white tie event:

This is the occasion which, unless she has a bottomless pit of cash, strikes anxiety or at least uncertainty into most women's hearts. Dresses fit for such events are not reasonably priced, so consider borrowing (if you can) a gown from a friend or female family member before searching for a new one to buy. Consider also purchasing a second hand dress from an online market place. There are a few dress agencies that can loan you a dress for a small fee, but this will depend on your location. If you must purchase your own for such a Cinderella moment, take the advice above concerning the Little Black Dress to avoid spending money on something you are unlikely to wear often. It may be kinder to your purse and your nerves if you restrain yourself from buying something *currently* fashionable in style or colour, or with very distinct print or embellishments. Choosing a gown so memorable and attention grabbing makes it *obvious* when you wear it again. There is nothing wrong with repeating a gown, but for the sake of feeling happy to attend another event in the same one, a plain, silk, satin, or taffeta dress may be more advantageous. You can always use a classic dress as a *base* and accessorise *around* it.

- Gowns must reach to the ankle or just skim the floor, purchase your shoes first (or wear a height similar to the shoe you will wear) when trying gowns to ensure the length is correct.

- Plain silk, taffeta or crepe gowns are the most versatile. Avoid prints and embellishments if you wish to re-use the gown. Velvets and damasks are nice for winter events, but inappropriate in finer weather.

- Gowns can be sleeveless but not strappy. Sleeves of any length are acceptable.

- The shape or outline of any undergarments should be completely undetectable.

- White tie events call for long gloves to the elbow or above it. They are worn at all times except for when dining.

- For formal events where there is to be dancing, wear your hair up if it is long and be careful of too much jewellery that dangles, it may prove a 'catching' hazard.

Skirts

"Why do women want to dress like men when they're fortunate enough to be women? Why lose femininity, which is one of our greatest charms? We get more accomplished by being charming than we would be flaunting around in pants and smoking. I'm very fond of men. I think they are wonderful creatures. I love them dearly. But I don't want to look like one. When women gave up their long skirts, they made a grave error".

This quote was written by children's author, illustrator, and vintage lifestyle enthusiast Tasha Tudor. Our modern outlook may initially recoil in horror at the obvious gender stereotyping, but think about it, we *do* have something that is rather special that adds a little charm to our style, not to mention is supremely useful in hot weather. Should we be celebrating the skirt more? Despite our hard work obtaining voting rights, equal career opportunities, and now borrowing from the wardrobes of boys, we are *still* able to keep hold of the beauty and charm of a feminine wardrobe, and cherish it if we wish. The skirt epitomises femininity, and though we may wish to wear trousers on occasion, the freedom and joy of wearing a skirt still belongs to women exclusively. Cool in summer, and freeing in winter when layered with tights to keep us warm and saving us from the prison of tight jeans, the skirt is actually one of the most comfortable and versatile pieces in our wardrobe. The anatomy of a good skirt is one which is flattering in shape and at a length comfortable for the individual. Etiquette and good taste however *does* dictate that a skirt should not be indecently short, ideally no shorter than just above the knee, or for that matter, too sheer. If you feel you would like to go shorter, try going wider in shape of the skirt first, the feeling of restriction in a long skirt can be remedied by a wider hemline. If you must go short then tights are your saving grace. Here are a few basic skirts that every woman should have in her wardrobe:

The **Country Skirt** is intended for leisure and weekend wear. Ideally knee length (just above or below) in a heavy cotton, boucle, denim chambray, tweed, wool, corduroy, moleskin, or suede it can look charming in winter paired with thick tights and boots. Skirts for the country do well in slightly a-lined shapes or at the very least are gored (several vertical panels sewn together), offering good width in the skirt at the knee for tromping over fields and stiles. It's no use restricting a woman's movement at the knee when cycling either. In winter and autumn, pair with knitwear over flannel shirts and blouses, in finer weather lighter blouses and sleeveless shell tops with cardigans. A lovely variation on the country skirt (but offers little versatility) is the kilt. Choose your tartan of an appropriate clan based on the heritage or your surname. Or if left to fend for oneself, defer to the Queen and pick Royal Stewart or the more versatile Blackwatch.

Suppliers: *Cordings of Picadilly, The House of Bruar, Joules, Brora, Boden, Great Scotland, Edinburgh Woollen Mill, Really Wild.*

Suppliers of Kilts: *All previous suppliers mentioned plus; Locharron of Scotland, Celtic & Co, Kinloch Anderson.*

Summer Skirts are when the ease, lightness, and sheer joy of being able to wear a skirt really comes into its own. Light cottons, cotton lawn, linen, chambray, and jersey will keep you delightfully cool. The options available for print, colour, embellishment and design are so widely varied it is wise to start with a capsule of skirts in basic colours and styles to match many outfits that you can pull out year after year, before you branch into fun and fashionable styles. A knee length, a-line chambray skirt and a light and darker linen skirt (one in stone and one in navy) will see you through most events. After that, add to your collection with brighter colours from your colour family. When wearing lighter fabrics on the bottom half, ensure that they are opaque enough so as not to reveal the outline of your underwear. The lighter the shade, the heavier the fabric should be, or at the very least a fine cotton should be lined. A white cotton lawn in a singular layer will do little to hide the pattern of your knickers! Remember also that when it comes to skirts for hot-weather wear, elasticated waists and a slightly looser fit are your best friends.

Summer is also a lovely time of year to embrace the cotton **Maxi Skirt**, in England's unpredictable weather it offers protection from both the sun and the sudden rain showers or cooler breezes which can blow in from the Atlantic at a moment's notice. Keep the maxi wide enough to allow full movement of the legs, it's no use bandaging yourself up in a skirt too narrow to allow you to walk properly. Ensure the length doesn't drag on the floor. Hem it if necessary. Summer maxi skirts have a relatively short shelf life (in terms of quality and duration of wear) so the investment shouldn't be extortionate. Have fun with batik prints, sailor stripes, and all over floral prints in colours to suit you.

Light fabric summer skirts look best paired with flat or low-heeled sandals (that encase the feet enough to provide support), canvas espadrilles, slim canvas plimsolls, and ballet flats. Unless one is on holiday or in a very casual setting with little walking to do, avoid toe-post flip-flops for the sake of your foot health (they are also rarely flattering on anyone).

Suppliers: Joules, Boden, White Stuff, Seasalt, Marks & Spencer, Fat Face, Mistral, Poetry.

The **Party Skirt** is a wonderful piece to have in your arsenal for evening events that call for those 'in between' outfits that are neither too formal, nor relaxed, but still require a little fancy effort. They are a fail-safe plan for when you just don't know what to wear! A fuller shaped skirt in a midi or knee length in rich sumptuous fabrics like velvet, shimmering knits, satin, silk, or heavy cotton featuring beading, bold prints, sequins, and embellishments can dress up a fine knit polo neck or plain black silk camisole and cardigan combination for semi-casual dates, dinner parties, or visits to the theatre and art galleries. Choose a shape that flatters you at the waist and a length that looks equally pleasing with low conservative heels, and flat ballet slippers—this is usually a knee length. Party skirts are most likely worn in the colder months, so select yours in darker coloured fabrics that look flattering and match well with opaque tights. Summer party skirts are pretty with tulle, fine embroidery, broderie anglaise, and silk organza.

Suppliers: Boden, Hobbs, Coast, Jaeger, Marks & Spencer, Phase Eight, Whistles.

The **Smart Pencil Skirt** is an indispensable item for formal occasions such as interviews, daily office wear, meetings with solicitors and dressing for sombre events such as funerals. One classic black or dark navy pencil skirt in a quality fabric can work with anything from a blouse and cardigan or fine knit sweater, to a structured blazer for any imaginable formal day event. Choose a high quality suiting or wool fabric for maximum versatility and longevity, the greater the quality of fabric the better the formality and polish of your overall look. Like a good pair of tailored trousers, the tailored pencil skirt is an item not to scrimp on. Make sure yours is fully lined and the closure is as subtle as possible, ideally a concealed zip to keep the line of your skirt trim and unspoiled.

Suppliers: Hobbs, Jaeger, Reiss, Joseph, Jigsaw, Winser London, Hawes & Curtis.

Trousers

Ladies should *never* wear trousers… only kidding! Though we joke, there should be a little observance to the fact that women are now very quick to put aside classic garments that connect us to our femininity on a daily basis. The wearing of trousers is easy, little thought has to go into your whole outfit when one throws a pair of jeans on, but this casts aside the whole joy of dressing as a lady, it shouldn't just be reserved for special occasions. You don't have to subscribe to dresses and skirts for the rest of your life to be considered feminine or look like a lady, but do try to rely less on trousers, especially if, like me and countless other women you find it hard to find a flattering cut in trousers. Generally men only need to find a trouser to fit two parts of their anatomy, the waist and inside leg, whereas ladies have to consider the waist, the hip, the roundness of the bottom, the rise, the inside leg and the circumference of the upper *and* lower leg. Frankly it can be exhausting to find a comfortable and flattering fit, so we are therefore going to look at the very basics of a trouser collection to see you through a modest range of events and daily errands.

For **Jeans**, likewise with the advice given previously for gentlemen, your best bet is to head for the old and highly favoured brands who have been manufacturing garments in denim since the dawn of the twentieth century. You can choose a classic fit such as the Levi's 501 (essentially a unisex cut) which is actually rather flattering on a lady. They don't play around with pocket placement, embellishments, or cut and so what you buy once will likely be exactly the same when re-purchasing again in five years or more (yes, that's how long *real* jeans last). The propensity these days of fast fashion and non-specialist brands to offer low-rise jeans is neither comfortable, nor flattering. Consider second hand or worn-in denim if you like a vintage look, they come without the price tag associated with purchasing 'factory distressed' denim. A mid-rise straight leg jean is flattering on almost all body types, with darker washes considered most slimming. So far as the inside leg measurement, pay thought to whether you are likely to wear heels with your jeans. If so, buy a pair to flatter your heel height and turn up the hem once or twice when wearing with flats.

Skinny Jeans with a mid or high-rise are also flattering, especially when worn with casual country attire and tucked into boots, or with sandals and loose blouses in milder weather. A little bit of stretch will help them keep their shape and stay form-fitting but stay away from *too* much stretch as these are likely to sag at the knee or bottom.

Remember: when you find a flattering pair of jeans that you love, buy as many pairs as you can afford. Fashionable 'fast fashion' denim styles, washes and cuts rarely repeat themselves season after season. A pair of jeans worn and washed regularly will offer you at most, twelve months of wear before they begin to look tired. Put aside this concern if you stick to long-standing heritage designs such as the 501 as they will always be available. Though the initial price may be dearer, the cost per wear will offer you better value in the long run.

Suppliers: *Levi, Lee, Wrangler.*

Moleskin & Corduroy Trousers are lovely casual items to wear when off-duty but a smarter-than-jeans look is desired. They are also beautifully warm and appropriate in autumn and winter, they elevate a look from being considered too casual. Paired with Chelsea boots or leather loafers they make for great weekend wear and are so much more flattering and mature than denim. Select cuts in a mid-rise with a straight leg for a classic look. Country colours look best in moleskin and corduroy fabrics, they exercise a 'borrowed from the boys look' and match with the Mr in shades of evergreen, mulberry, navy, ochre, and chocolate. Pair with country shirts and cable knits.

Suppliers: The House of Bruar, Orvis, Land's End, R.M. Williams, Country Collections.

Slacks, or Classic Tailored Trousers are generally reserved for work wear and are paired with lightweight shell tops or blouses in summer, to chunkier knitwear in winter. Alongside the classic pencil skirt, purchase yours in the best quality and tailoring you can afford. The preference of the shape of the cut is individual, but to ensure good versatility and being appropriate, keep them mid-rise or above. Not only are lower cut trousers uncomfortable, they are not appropriate for the office as they expose too much of the lower back and sometimes the top of the bottom! They also never offer themselves up for the tucking in of blouses and shirts very nicely. Trousers with a waistband that sits at the smallest part of your waist (usually labeled as high-waisted) is the most flattering cut for a woman. Classic straight leg trousers and cigarette pants look nice with courts and loafers, while a wide leg in a gorgeously draped suiting or wool look stunning when paired with court shoes or heeled boots. Consider black for your first pair, then add to your wardrobe with a dark navy, air force blue, or dark grey flannel for variety and a softer look. Ladies working in creative environments can play with prints and much brighter colours.

Suppliers: Hobbs, L.K. Bennett, Reiss, Jaeger, Austin Reed, Whistles, Jigsaw, Winser London, Boden, Baukjen, Hawes & Curtis, Karen Millen.

Summer Trousers usually come in the guise of **Linen** or a cropped **Capri** in a light Tencel or medium-weight cotton. Ensure, as with lighter summer skirts, that they provide adequate opacity, and ideally are elasticated or adjustable at the waist for maximum comfort. Ladies have a lot of flexibility with summer trousers in contrast to the male of the species, but that does not mean quality should suffer for the sake of fashion. Linen has a tendency to fade in colour, and after repeated wear and washing, especially when artificially dyed. Stick to natural flax tones for greater shelf-life. Polyester and Tencel trousers are beautifully lightweight, but can lack in breathability. Favour an elastic panel in the waist for maximum comfort, with wider and looser cuts in the leg. Whether you are comfortable wearing **Shorts** is a matter of personal taste, but for etiquette's sake steer clear of 'short-shorts'. The bottom hem of the short should sit at the mid-thigh, not the crease of the buttock! Cut-off denim is the reserve of fit young surf-types, even then they aren't particularly becoming or elegant, and definitely not appropriate for anywhere but the beach. **Chino** style trousers and shorts are flattering and offer a smart-casual solution on home-shores and abroad. Sport shorts are worn for *playing* sports. **Leggings** too are only appropriate for sportswear or layering with pieces such as a tunic or dress that *entirely* covers the bottom and groin area. Too many times have women unknowingly flashed a bad pair of knickers or a camel-toe to onlookers due to the weave of their leggings being stretched so thin— yikes.

Suppliers: White Stuff, Seasalt, Crew Clothing, Boden, Gap, Gant, Poetry, Jigsaw.

Knitwear

For classic woollen sweaters, to pair with skirts, trousers and wear over blouses and country shirts, the **Aran Sweater** or **Guernsey** are beautiful options. Another alternative made from cotton instead of a wool-based knit is a **Breton**. Ladies should ideally source theirs from the ladies and families who still knit these icons of British design by hand, most offer both unisex and female specific patterns and designs. The history and particulars of each item mentioned can be found in the gentleman's knitwear section of this book.

Suppliers: Guernsey Woollens , Blarney Woollen Mills, Old Harry.

For quality **Fine Knitwear** such as the crew or v-neck pullover, vest, or polo neck in merino wool, cashmere or lambswool in similar styles look lovely worn alone (with a camisole or thermal vest underneath), or over a collared blouse, office appropriate or country shirt. They can be paired with most separates in the wardrobe.

Suppliers: Johnstons of Elgin, Orvis, Brora, The House of Bruar, Ralph Lauren, Crew Clothing, Edinburgh Woollen Mill.

Cardigans are versatile and very feminine. They look charming paired with dresses and over blouses with skirts. Provided it is an acceptable setting, they can also look smart in the workplace. Finer gauge knits are suitable for work, while longer line cardigans and chunky knits are best for casual and weekend wear.

Suppliers: *The House of Bruar, Mistral, Cordings of Picadilly, WoolOvers, Boden, White Stuff, Denner Cashmere.*

Notes on natural fibre knitwear: Natural fibres cannot be beaten for quality, warmth and authenticity to an English inspired wardrobe. Though the care requires specific washing instructions, detergents and storage, acrylic knitwear just cannot compare. Not only do natural fibres allow your skin to breathe, they feel luxurious and won't attract static like acrylic. Invest in a good wool detergent, a pill-comb and cedar blocks to keep your knits protected and looking beautiful. There are lovely cotton and hemp sweaters available if you are investing in an animal compassionate wardrobe.

Sports, fleeces, and novelty sweaters

Ladies can look lovely in 'permanently borrowed' **Sports Jerseys** or **College Rugby Tops,** likely stolen from the husband. It is the ultimate big comfy sweater for off-duty wear, nicely coupled with a pair of jeans, plimsolls, or thrown on with wellies in order to walk the dog.

Suppliers: *Your husband's wardrobe, Ryder & Amies, Crew Clothing, Hackett London, or official college and sporting stores.*

Fleeces are an easy way to keep out the chill and a clear favourite of the farmer's wife and equestrian set. There is nothing particularly ladylike or elegant about them, but it cannot be denied they pay their way in English winters—stick with the recommended manufacturers.

Suppliers: *Schöffel, Patagonia, Barbour, Musto.*

Sweatshirts are, by and large, an obvious way to tell people where you shop, which is very unbecoming. Branding, Disney characters, slogans, and the like will only serve you for a season or so. Therefore invest little if your budget is little. A traditionally elegant English lady is unlikely to wear what is known as a *sweat*shirt unless she is heading to the gym, under the weather, expecting no company, or scrubbing her bathroom.

Suppliers: *Vintage clothing dealers, or sporting stores.*

Tennis, or Cricket Jumpers are as classic as they come and another great item to 'borrow from the boys'. Featuring a v-neck in a deeply ribbed or cable knit with long sleeves, or sleeveless, the Cricket jumper is synonymous with traditional English sporting style. Always in a shade of white or cream wool with one or two bands (to match your college, sports team or regiment colours), along the neckline, and sometimes wrist or waistband. Wear yours over a cotton dress or pair with a floaty maxi skirt to keep out the chill on an overcast summer's day. Like the boys, you can pair yours with jeans and plimsolls for a casual air.

Suppliers: His wardrobe, Luke Eyres of Cambridge, Smart Turnout London, Peter Christian, Rochford Sports.

The same advice given to the gentlemen regarding **Novelty Sweaters** applies to the ladies as well; they are wickedly entertaining at Christmas, with cheeky slogan knits being a particular favourite with fashion influencers, celebrities, (and even old dukes). *Always* wear yours with nonchalance without any expectation of being taken seriously. Occasional forays into silly knitwear is unexpected and cuts a quirky dash in an otherwise serious reputation, but consistent wear is a little childish if not worn on the right occasion. They are never appropriate for work and watch out for the 'message' you are sending out, especially in the playground—some slogans can be inappropriate. Know your moments. The exception to this rule is what is known as the *Intarsia* sweater. You *can* look cute with a sausage dog or love hearts incorporated into the knit on your jumper, just keep them for weekend wear.

Suppliers: Joules, Boden, Cath Kidston, Baukjen.

The best thing about women's knitwear is that sometimes it really is best (and perfectly acceptable) to **borrow from the boys.** Nothing beats that feeling of overwhelming comfort and joy when putting on an over-sized jumper to walk the dog or slum around the house than when it has been stolen—sorry, 'permanently borrowed'—from your husband, boyfriend, brother, or dad.

Tops, shirts, and blouses

Blouses, shell tops and camisoles create a sea of separates in any woman's wardrobe. It is overwhelming to even think about describing all the options available. So what makes a classic, and which should you concentrate your efforts and budget on? High street designers churn out different cuts, patterns, colours, and themes season after season, so we shall look at the *reigning* classics and what make up a good capsule wardrobe of separate pieces. Ones which co-ordinate nicely with skirts, slacks and jeans. Forget not the colours and tones that you suit you, disregard what is fashionable right now and look for quality that lasts.

The **Classic White Shirt or Blouse** is indispensable for a woman's working wardrobe as well as for leisure. Depending on the occasion for which you wish to wear it, the material of a white blouse or shirt can take you from court to camping. For formal use, choose beautiful flowing silks (requiring greater care), or fine crisp cottons. A ladies version of the **Oxford Cloth Button Down** is equally lovely for work and weekend as they offer modesty and smartness due to the durability of the cloth and the classic styling, but can instantly be dressed down for wearing untucked with a rolled sleeve. White, light blues, and pinks are widely available, while some shirt makers offer prints, ginghams, stripes, and windowpane prints for the working and weekend wardrobe. **Linen Shirts** and gauzy crepes are best kept for the weekend. Pay special attention to the structure and tailoring of a shirt or blouse to deem whether it is appropriate for work. Blouses worn to the office should be as minimal in embellishment, loud prints and 'styling' as possible with no trailing sleeves, fiddly bits, or ties. Some English country women have been known to borrow their husband's shirts for weekend pursuits—a worn-in billowing men's shirt loosely tucked into a skirt or jeans and rolled at the sleeves can look very pretty when off-duty.

Suppliers LilySilk, Hawes & Curtis, Crew Clothing, The House of Bruar, Joules, Ralph Lauren, Reiss, Jaeger, Hobbs, L.K. Bennett, T.M. Lewin, MiaGiacca, Really Wild.

The **Tattersall or Country Shirt** is a useful and quintessential item for an English country wardrobe. They pair nicely with smarter moleskin trousers or country skirts and for layering underneath knitwear, a fleece, or padded gilet. Tattersall shirts consist of a large or small gridded pattern over the fabric in two or more complementary colours. Making them very easy to pair with different items in the wardrobe and were originally inspired by the blankets worn by thoroughbreds at Newmarket. Being so synonymous with country and equestrian wear, the colours making up the checks are often muted in natural shades on a cream or neutral background, but more adventurous colours such as purples and bright neons can now be found. Country shirt designers offer lovely ladies shirts in plaids, tartans, brushed cottons, or all-over motifs such as pheasants, hares, and racehorses. These look really nice paired with jeans for a weekend in the country.

Suppliers: Cordings of Piccadilly, Rydale, The House of Bruar, Orvis, Barbour, Musto, Purdey.

Oh the **Plain T-shirt**, such a basic thing to need, such a hard thing to find in good quality. The quest to find the perfect white tee in a cut that is flattering, washes well, and doesn't twist at the seams is like finding a needle in a haystack. The modus operandi when sourcing and purchasing this wardrobe basic is to consider how much you are willing to pay for perfection. There are a select few retailers who claim they make the best, but you must define for *yourself* what you consider that to be. You can walk into any supermarket these days and pick up a basic t-shirt for under a fiver, but it probably won't last you all that long, and you likely won't love it. If you demand a nicer quality and experience for something that you wear so consistently, then consider looking at *ethical and sustainable* clothing companies, their focus is mainly on constructing quality basic pieces that are incomparable when it comes to wash and wear. They can't be flamboyant when it comes to design or manufacturing so have to make the absolute best of the basics they *can* produce. Bamboo has had a lot of good press in recent years as a beautifully soft alternative to cotton that has a wonderful drape, is breathable, and hypoallergenic. Purchasing your basics in materials such as these (especially as we go through many of them in our lifetime), can be a unique way to make a difference. Consider also purchasing from manufacturers who use strictly organic cotton.

Suppliers: *Thought Clothing, Rapanui, Dharma Bums, BAM Bamboo Clothing, Poetry, Positive Outlook, Boody, Seasalt.*

The extension to your basic t-shirt category is the **Jersey or Striped Breton** top, so useful for weekend wear the Breton style has become somewhat of a classic with a resurgence in the last decade or so. They are usually found in a three quarter length sleeve and made of a slightly thicker weight jersey. They wash and wear very well.

Suppliers: *Joules, Boden, Seasalt, Crew Clothing, White Stuff, Fat Face, The Breton Shirt Co, The Nautical Company.*

For casual summer days, a **Pique Polo Shirt** pairs well with casual cotton or denim skirts, shorts and cropped trousers. The short sleeves and open collar keep you cool and comfortable but look smart in comparison to a basic t-shirt. White is a classic colour, but can look a little 'school uniform'. There are a variety of pastels and vibrant colours available from classic retailers of the polo shirt.

Suppliers: *Fred Perry, Lacoste, Joules, Crew Clothing.*

There are plenty of other shirt and blouse types available in womenswear. Once you have the basics covered you can further add to your wardrobe according to taste and style. However you must remember that in order to curate a classic English wardrobe it must be immune to whim and wholly practical before all things. Consider the practicality and versatility of an item, and how classic a piece is *before* it wins a place in your closet. Will it match with what you already have? It's no use going mad for sparkles, chiffon, and sequins in one season if all you do is muck out horses and herd the kids to and from school. Keeping an eye on trends and pining after them without much thought to whether or not these items will suit *your* lifestyle is a certain way to waste money and leave you dissatisfied, feeling like you have nothing to wear.

Coats and Jackets

Proper **Raincoats** you would think, are a non-negotiable item to have in England, however it would appear that many ladies find favour in soaking through a down jacket instead of opting for suitable protection from the rain. Many brands offer lightweight and nicely styled 'slickers' in pretty prints and bright colours. The key to a good raincoat is the fabric. For optimum weatherproofing look for rubberised cotton, or weatherproofed IsoTex. Choosing a lighter weight, non-bulky raincoat which can be worn over layers or happily carried when not in use, is the ideal investment as it will see you through many seasons. They can be worn over fleece and heavy sweaters as well as lighter skirts and dresses, and not look *as* out of place as a down jacket would in fairer weather rainstorms. For a classic look, opt for a full length navy, or hunter green for country wear and the ultimate protection from rain— superb for dog walking. Such classic styling will stand the test of time and gives off a 'hardier' and authentic look in the country, as if you are part of the furniture. Town dwellers who are likely to get caught in inclement weather during school runs, errands, and commuting around town may wish to opt for a three-quarter length jacket that sits just below the hip, of which colour and styling options are personal preference. Brighter saturated colours and fun prints are good for the school run, offering high visibility.

Suppliers: Joules, Boden, Seasalt, Stutterheim, Country Collections, The House of Bruar.

The iconic **Trench Coat**, sometimes referred to as a **Macintosh** is a smarter option for rainwear and pairs particularly well with business attire or when one wishes to wear an outfit with heels. Made of cotton gabardine, a lightweight but breathable waterproof fabric, one purchased loose enough to wear over a suit or smarter outfit can elevate your look better than a slicker. The classic design of a trench or 'mac' includes a double breasted ten button closure, epaulettes, raglan sleeves, a storm and gun flap, and is belted at the waist. Modern designs often do away with the 'additions' of storm flaps and epaulettes, instead streamlining the look leaving just the double-breasted closure and a belt for cinching at the waist. A traditional length is below the knee to mid-calf (though shorter hip length styles are available), and usually khaki or camel in colour, though navy, green, and red are now very fashionable too. Many fast fashion designers release this design in the autumn but fail to hit the mark on true durability or weatherproofing.

Suppliers: If you wish to invest in a true trench or macintosh to last you a lifetime, look to Aquascutum, or Burberry, both noted for their loyalty to the original design and superior finishes. For modestly priced options look at Hobbs or Jaeger.

A classic **Waxed Jacket** is synonymous with English country living, makers of the finest are the unrivalled J. Barbour & Sons. No country woman's wardrobe for dog walking, shooting, or outdoor pursuits is complete without a waxed jacket. Ignore the company's recent diversion toward dressing the 'trendy crowd' and source yours from a specialised country clothing outfitters who will supply *original* styles suitable for country wear. Forget looking at the range for women and instead go straight to the classic Beaufort and Bedale, they are sold as 'mens' but offer a true country fit. Hardy English countrywomen care not for waist definition or form-fitting styles unless they wish them to appear 'fashionable', at which point the proper reason for wearing a waxed jacket is lost. Waxed jackets are treated in Sylkoil making the fabric both weather and thorn proof. A well cared for waxed Barbour will last you a lifetime if you maintain it. Rewaxing once a year will keep it in good order. Barbour offer a rewax, repair and alteration service for a nominal fee should you require it.

Suppliers: Barbour.

Another coat for country and weekend wear is the **Quilted Coat**. A perfect companion in chilly weather, a quilted coat can offer warmth and style in a more flattering way than traditional weatherproof garments. Quilting has an equestrian look and pairs rather nicely with jeans and boots. Most quilted coats are now designed to sit at hip length with belts or self-cinched styling at the waist to nip you in and flatter the figure, however a proper country coat has a rather boxier shape intended for wearing over many layers. Quilted vests are another option for in between seasons and look fine with knitwear and jersey Breton tops. The Queen has been known to wear her quilted jackets off-duty, visiting at country shows, and while inspecting her horses. Keep yours for similar pursuits and choose classic navy or olive green with a cord collar, diamond pattern stitching and press stud closure.

Suppliers: Barbour, Joules, Musto, Crew Clothing, Regatta.

The **Blazer** is a gorgeous lightweight jacket option for the fairer months in suiting or linen, or if styled in heavier materials, great for layering under outerwear when you wish to look smarter than one would just wearing a sweater. The **Suiting Blazer**, classic in navy or black, is a great way to dress up a blouse worn with jeans or slacks and heels for office and casual wear. A blazer also pairs nicely with flowing silk dresses, offering more warmth than a cardigan.

The **Wool Blazer** can also achieve the same smart-casual effect while a **Boucle Jacket**, oft taking inspiration from Chanel is smarter still. **Country Tweed Blazers** are lovely for dressing up casual country-wear such as denim or moleskin jeans and dark brown boots, even a silk or flowing cotton skirt paired with tights, a jumper and wellies! The menswear equivalent of the women's blazer is known as the **Sport Jacket**, a design akin to a formal blazer but intended to be worn *without* matching trousers (which would make it a suit). While the men's styles are often looser or 'sack like' in cut with little or no shaping to the waist, women's styles are cut close to the body, with some featuring soft shoulder pads to define the shape even further. The corduroy jackets, tweeds, wools, and linen jackets you find in womenswear are a relaxed cousin to the more formal blazer that you would wear to work or a formal event. The sport coat is better suited to off-duty wear or casual work environments. They are usually single breasted with one of two button closures, narrow lapels, and feature no breast pocket, but patch front pockets are often seen. Wear a casual sport blazer with chinos, jeans, and moleskin trousers, or light flowing dresses. They look lovely when layered over a blouse or Oxford shirt and lightweight knit. Navy wool suiting blazers look fantastic paired with Breton stripe jerseys, jeans, and plimsolls too. The aim when finding a sport jacket is to pick one in a colour, cut, and fabric to suit the majority of your wardrobe for dress up and dress down days.

Suppliers: Smythe, Crew Clothing, Joules, L.K. Bennett, Whistles, Hobbs, MiaGiacci, Cordings of Piccadilly, Country Casuals, Jaeger, Joseph, Reiss, Peter Hahn, Gant, Boden, The House of Bruar, Really Wild.

A classic heavy **Wool Overcoat** is the backbone of a winter wardrobe for both ladies and gentlemen. In womenswear we refer to the overcoat as a single or double breasted cashmere or heavy wool coat to be worn on smart occasions. Tweeds and herringbones can also provide a stylish but still warm alternative. The classic overcoat is knee length or longer with flap or jetted pockets, is fully lined, and makes a very elegant and classic staple in a woman's wardrobe. They lend unrivalled warmth and provide a stylish and conservative look where 'down jackets' and weatherproofed coats do not. When looking for a wool overcoat choose a classic colour such as black, navy, or camel.

Necklines that are high, or at least able to be buttoned up provide better protection against the cold. Many woollen overcoats are cut close to the body with shaping and often belts at the waist. Pick a size that is comfortable enough when you layer a lightweight blazer or thick jumper underneath. Woollen coats look better for formal workwear and events than the type of coats you may pick for casual weekends. They are certainly an investment, but a wool or cashmere coat well stored and cared for should last for decades, which is why it is best to plump for a classic look over something trendy.

Look also for Wool **Pea Coats, or Reefer Coats** for casual shorter styles and to don in cool weather. An equally warm coat with achingly classic styling that takes the formality down a notch is the **Duffle Coat**. A firm favourite of Paddington Bear and synonymous with English school-years, this icon is well worth having in your collection. Choose from camel, charcoal, navy, or a beautiful deep red for that Great British look.

Suppliers: The House of Bruar, Hobbs, Boden, L.K. Bennett, Marks & Spencer, Gant, Jaeger, Reiss, Jigsaw, Brora.
For Duffle & Pea Coats: *Gloverall, Original Montgomery.*

For beautiful formal events or for the want of wearing something exquisite, nothing but a **Frock Coat** will do. These are a complete luxury and require much consideration before purchase, as it is likely you will only need or own one in your lifetime. They are a little hard (but not impossible) to find on the general high street, but if you'd like to design your own frock coat it is a good idea to source a tailor or bespoke designer who can create something for you that is not only made perfectly for your shape but will flatter your skin tone and current wardrobe too. The frock coat is essentially a work of art, featuring frogging, intricate tapestry stitching or quilting, embroidery, beading or detailed and unique hand block printing. Usually plain and streamlined in cut, of velvet, linen, jacquard, or shantung silk fabric, the detailing and beauty of a frock coat is found in the decoration. The ideal length is between mid-thigh to just below the knee, allowing you to wear it with tailored slacks, jeans, and a formal dress. Many ladies who own frock coats like to pair theirs with turn-ups and plimsolls too, the key is to *own it* and embrace the attention and compliments that such a highly decorative piece of clothing will bring you. They certainly stand out from the crowd, and they rightly deserve to.

Suppliers: Beatrice Von Tresckow, Madeleine, Monsoon, Toast, Nomads Clothing, Monsoon, Shibumi, Moloh, Really Wild, Katherine Hooker.

Hats, fascinators, and hair accessories

Where once stood a generation of women who wouldn't be caught dead leaving the house without a hat, now we have a generation who only seem to slap on a chapeau when the temperatures plummet. Hats and hair accessories offer such an exciting way to personalise any outfit, and so many of us are missing out on that joy. Nice hats can be so incredibly elegant, feminine, and they look very respectful. It's hard to be ignored in a good hat!

While not all styles are suitable for your face shape, experimenting will soon help you to find the styles that suit your features as well as your lifestyle. Listed below are hats that you can wear daily to elevate your look and keep your head warm or shielded from the sun.

A quick word on hair; we've all probably been the victims of 'hat hair' at some point, and there are a few things you can do to navigate the issue:

- Make sure the headband is not too tight, a close fitting band may leave a dent in your hair and forehead. Get a hat that fits, you should be able to comfortably put a finger between the hat and your head.
- Ensure your hair is *fully* dry before you put a hat on.
- If you have a fringe, part it gently, or brush to one side before putting on a hat. Then correct it and brush back into place when you remove the hat.
- Tuck your hair behind your ears. Pressure from the hat is concentrated around the brow and temples so keeping hair out of the way avoids, creases, dents and bumps.
- If your hair has a wavy or curly texture, gently scrunch your hair up a little before putting the hat on so that it does not drag the hair down and create an unnatural looking straight section.
- Know your materials. Coarse textured wool hats will create greater friction and leave more indents and frizz than a fine cashmere.
- Don't be tempted to brush your hair right away as it may cause static and frizz. Try finger combing before reaching for a brush.
- Dry shampoo or a little texturing paste may help revive hair that has gone limp.
- If you have long hair, carry a hairband or large grip and create a messy up-do when you remove your hat indoors. No one will know the difference.
- For formal events such as weddings or funerals opt for a sleek low chignon hairstyle or half-up do and use a pin to keep your hat secure. Loose hairstyles that fall in the face will look messy and are harder to 'rescue' once you remove your hat.

- If all else fails, adopt a laissez-faire attitude, roll with it and laugh it off—no one is immune to hat hair.

Winter Hats, believe it or not, are available in more styles and shapes than just the bobble hat or the beanie. While cute for the deepest of freezes and quick errands, they aren't always the most stylish of options, especially if you are faced with the dilemma of having to dress up when the temperatures drop. A lovely option for smart day wear, the **Cloche Hat** is not so wide in the brim that you feel like you are wearing a statement hat, because they fit so close to the head and the brim profile is small and slightly down-turned they do not catch on windy days. Cloche hats come in a variety of winter colours in wool, they look best paired with tailored wool coats and gabardine trench coats. Cloche hats can also sometimes be found in straw for summer wear and look very pretty with floaty dresses, giving off a 'Lady Mary' feel from the 1930s. A **Pillbox Hat** is also a nice choice for a modest, slimline, and unassuming hat which still looks stylish for formal occasions.

Suppliers: Christy's Hats, Lock & Co, Marks & Spencer.

Flat crown hats which serve most casual outfits well and also tolerate a bit of 'wear and tear' such as folding, rolling, and stuffing into a handbag are the **Beret, Flat Cap, Baker Boy & Breton** (also known as a fisherman's or mariner's cap). Classic wool beret hats come in a vast array of colours and are often moderately priced, so a collection to match most outfits is achievable. A modest set consisting of black, navy, red, and camel should match almost all outfits and occasions. The Breton cap looks great with a nautical themed outfit, choose yours in a navy/black wool or weatherproofed cotton. The flat cap and baker boy are made for country tweed or tartan wool and so look best when worn with a country outfit and quilted or waxed jacket. These styles tend to sit quite tightly around the circumference of the head and so offer little space for hair to pile under the hat, they also refuse to co-operate with a high ponytail. Pull hair into a low style or wear it loose. The beret is the only flat hat that is transferable to smarter settings, leave all others for weekend or leisure outfits. Consider also looking to men's outfitters for these styles, they generally offer classic designer pieces compared to those on offer at 'fashion forward' stores that adopt sub-standard methods of production.

Suppliers: Village Hats, Christy's Hats, Lock & Co, Cordings of Piccadilly, Barbour, Alan Paine, Dubarry.

There are many wonderful companies now producing very realistic, but thankfully very faux, **Fur Hats, Headbands & Earmuffs**. Prepare to defend yourself with a good argument if you support the fur trade, national tolerance is very low. Shades of black, ivory, and vibrant jewel colours look stunning with winter tailoring for smart evening wear or weddings, and muted 'real' looking *dappled* furs look great with country jackets, boots, and tweed. Be mindful of wearing fur in the rain or very wet misty weather as it can go limp very quickly. Faux fur looks charming in the snow, just make sure to brush any flakes of snow away as soon as you are indoors so they don't melt into the fabric, then hang your hat to air dry before storing. Real fur when wet will smell of soggy doggies. Another reason to go faux.

Suppliers: Dubarry, The House of Bruar, Helen Moore, or vintage (for real fur).

A ladies **Country Hat** is indispensable in the British Isles. Unless one wishes to don a transparent rain hood, good options for keeping you dry are the **Waxed Bucket** hat, usually offering a down turned brim, ruching on the crown, and is heavily waterproofed. They are soft in construction, usually crushable and good to have in the pocket of a raincoat or stashed somewhere in the car. The bucket rain hat is a casual option, but for those looking for something smarter, a **Waxed Bushman** may be a more stylish example. Modelled on a style similar to the wool felt **Fedora**, they make stunning country wear for walks, pub lunches, and even smart enough for the races (when you attend for the sport, not the drunkenness). Many hat makers are now embellishing the fedora and bushman hat with lovely country motifs such as feathers, braided leather ribbons, spent shotgun cartridges, and buckles.

Suppliers: Christy's Hats, Cordings of Piccadilly, Barbour, Lock & Co, The House of Bruar, Cotswold Country Hats.

Knitted **Beanie & Bobble Hats** are a dime a dozen, but if you are looking for something a bit special than your usual supermarket or fast fashion offering, look on Etsy for knitters who sell beautiful handcrafted Arans, Fair Isles and hats knitted from vintage patterns. Many take custom orders so you can find something to suit your style and colour preferences. If you'd prefer something off the peg, then visit an outfitter that caters to the 'outdoor' lifestyle. Their offerings have often been vigorously tested for wear and reviewed in all sorts of weather conditions. For around the same price as a basic hat from a fast fashion store you'll end up with something that does what it promises, keeping you warm!

Suppliers: Barts, The North Face, Go Outdoors, Blacks, Mountain Warehouse, The House of Bruar, or Etsy for hand knit items.

Summer Hats are where the fun really begins for a lady. Where winter hats are worn for mostly practical reasons, a sun hat is not only practical for keeping out the sun but adds such a lovely charm to a daily outfit regardless of the formality of the events you attend, and places frequented. In fact, formality and whether you hat will be appropriate is a thought you can set aside while the swifts and swallows are in residence. If you choose only one, stick with a daily straw hat. The National Health Service heavily suggest you 'slap on a hat', so why wouldn't you?

The classic **Wide Brim Straw Hat** is most appropriate for almost any occasion during the warmer months. Simple styles with neutral grosgrain ribbons or self-fabric bows look equally lovely with a light dress and cardigan, or casual t-shirt and shorts. If you want to dress up a straw hat for a wedding or garden party event, simply add fresh flowers, or faux flowers in the form of a pin or brooch. A stiffer brimmed hat will look better for formal events over the casual 'floppy' daily sun hat you'd tend to the garden in. It's a good idea to buy a plain formal straw hat and invest in a rainbow of ribbons and accessories to swap out and match with your outfit for versatility.

Suppliers of ribbons: V.V. Rouleaux, MacCulloch & Wallis.

For style statements, the straw **Panama, Fedora & Boater** are dressier versions of the standard straw hat with distinctive brims and shapes. They look charming but tend to sway toward a more formal or 'considered' look. They look great for events and days where you have made an effort with your outfit, but sometimes out of place on a Saturday morning strolling at the farmer's market. Choose genuine handwoven Panamas from Ecuador, the 'Montechristi' model being the most exclusive and luxurious, some taking up to four months to weave. The Planter Panama is an elegant and distinctive style with a round flat brim and changeable brim bands, most synonymous with sugar plantation workers and river boatman on the Mississippi. The classic boater (or Skimmer as sometimes known), crafted from stiff sisal straw and topped with a band of petersham ribbon offers a traditionally English summer look perfect for punting, picnics, and barbecues.

Suppliers: Lock & Co, Christy's Hats, Gamble & Gunn, Village Hats, The Panama Hat Company.

The **Cotton Sun Hat**, sometimes known as **Bucket Hats** are for the most casual of days and events. They are styled similar to a cloche with a down turned brim which is often flipped up at the forehead. Many are machine washable, and some reversible offering a plain or patterned design. Bucket hats are designed to be crushable, so are great for traveling and stashing in the car. They are not considered stylish enough for formal events, but are a prettier version for those who would usually consider a baseball cap (which, unless she is playing sport or doing manual labour, the English rose would not consider wearing). The **Straw Visor** is a more feminine option to the baseball cap, it offers shade to the eyes but little protection to the crown of the head. A linen or cotton **Safari Hat** is a cool, country option styled similar to a fedora or bushman.

For sun hats in cotton or straw look also to the brands and shops catering to men. They have a variety of styles in plain, conservative, and highly classic options not usually offered to women (our choices are usually a bit more fashionable and trendy according to the style of the season). After all a head size is just a head size. Borrow from the boys!

Suppliers: *Village Hats, Etsy, Orvis, Wallaroo.*

Funeral hats

Please do refrain from veils and flamboyant funeral hats unless you are the grieving widow. Such a *display* of grief is not very English and has been largely glamorised by old Hollywood movies. A veil at a funeral is not correct, neither is a hat with much decoration. Look to the female members of the royal family and study what they wear for Remembrance Sunday. The design needs to be as restrained as possible, in nothing but black on black. The closest acceptable colour is the darkest of navy. Wool and felt are appropriate fabrics. Brims are allowed, but nothing *too* wide. The design and shaping needs to be conservative and nothing should draw attention to any aspect of the hat or block another person's view. A fail-safe option which can be worn for other events is a cloche hat. Let it be said that a dark hat for a funeral in the height of summer is not de rigueur. Instead, keep your hairstyle polished and conservative. If you must accessorise your hair, a black headband or ribbon to tie a ponytail is pretty. An umbrella or parasol instead of a hat can be useful to shield you from the sun during a burial. Never wear a fascinator to a funeral.

Hat etiquette at funerals:

- It is no longer deemed customary to wear a hat, unless you wish to or are expected to by family members, the choice to wear one is yours.
- You are there to honour the deceased, this is not a time to make a fashion statement.
- Ideally no outlandish feathers, embellishment or flowers. Velvet, grosgrain, or matte satin ribbons acceptable but only 'tone on tone'.

- Do not wear anything that will obstruct the view of people sat behind you during the remembrance service.
- Veils are reserved for the widow and the closest female family members only.
- If the service is to be held in a religious service different to what you are used to, research or ask what is appropriate (hats may not be so).
- Keep your hat on for the funeral service and for the burial or cremation.
- Remove your hat at the wake.

Suppliers: Lock & Co Hatters, Christy's London, Jaxon & James.

Wedding hats

Much like hats for funerals, unless one is attending a 'society' or royal wedding, the wearing of hats to weddings has lost popularity. When things are no longer *expected* laziness tends to rears its ugly head. True, the wearing of a hat and co-ordinating an outfit to match is an effort, but when else can a lady have so much fun truly dressing up? It's not as though we all walk a red carpet every weekend.

We must make a greater effort to keep milliners in business. If expense is your concern then find a hat agency in your local area. For a small fee (or at least smaller than that of a very expensive hat) you can rent a good hat for the weekend. They tend to have a variety from many different designers so you can be sure to find something to suit almost any outfit and flatter any face. If you would like to purchase your own hat, consider starting your collection with a light cream shade in sinamay that will match with most pastels or lighter spring shades. Then add to your collection with a navy which will suit blues, deeper or vibrant pinks, reds, and yellows. After that the world is your oyster. Remember that weddings are not the same as a day at the races, though it is a nice excuse to dress up and make an effort, the attention should *not* be on you, but wholly on the bride.

Hat etiquette for weddings:

- Ensure that your hat does not create a distraction during the ceremony—no extra-wide brims or big trims that could block the view.
- Get your hair professionally styled (ideally fully up or at least half-up half-down) and the hat pinned and secured by a hairdresser.
- Visit an expert milliner or shop, they know which styles will suit your face, body frame, and height.

- Hats must be removed at, or shortly after 6pm. Ideally remove it soon after the speeches during the wedding breakfast (essentially after all formalities). This timely removal of a hat is why it is ideal to have hair professionally coiffured as the hairdresser will ensure you still look polished *under* the hat.
- Never outshine your hosts. The bride, her mother, and the mother of the groom should have the most attention grabbing hats. Keep yours classic and conservative.
- Fascinators are fun, but do not hold as much gravitas or elegance for a grown woman like a hat does. Much like tiara etiquette, if you are married opt for a hat and keep playful fascinators for the *much* younger set.

Suppliers: Rosie Olivia, William Chambers, Phase Eight, Whiteley Hats, or hat rental agencies.

Specialist Millinery is of course an option for you if your pockets are deep and you wish to match an outfit for an event exactly. A hat made especially for you is surely something to treasure, but as they make such a statement one should consider how many times you would get to wear it and whether it is worth the investment. I am in full support of the millinery trade but start your collection with the classics *first*, lest you be left with a wardrobe stuffed to the brim and "nothing to wear".

Tiaras, if worn as a serious fashion accessory, and not for fancy dress are reserved for brides or little girls playing dress-up. If you are lucky enough to own or inherit a *real* tiara (one never buys her own), then you will know that they are worn only by married women. This is correct etiquette for all levels of society. Blood princesses have sometimes been known to break the rules, borrow (from mummy) and wear them while yet unmarried, but the fiancée of a prince or duke will not don a tiara until those abbey bells ring for her. Tiaras are useful in that they serve as an obvious visual cue to refrain from approaching a lady romantically if her head is bedecked in diamonds or precious stones. Tiaras are only worn for the most formal of occasions, at dusk or later.

Hair accessories

Hair accessories for the grown woman are making somewhat of a comeback, namely the **Alice Band** and the **Velvet Hair Ribbon** which are the epitome of femininity. The English rose and any lady who takes style references from what we call the 'Sloaney Pony look' will know they never truly went away.

Any woman with hair longer than her jawline will find use from a modest wardrobe of hair accessories including the following:

- A matte satin or velvet Alice band in one of the regulation school colours, an inch wide. Black, navy, maroon, or emerald. One will do, lovely to have all four.
- A scrunchie, also in regulation school colours. Kinder on the hair than thin elastics, a hardy English rose is confident enough to wear out of doors, her shier sisters keep theirs for 'indoors'.
- A silk scarf to protect her crowning glory on country drives and windy weather. Knotted firmly under the chin, 'Granny chic' is practical and here to stay. Grace Kelly and the Queen made it cool.
- French barettes in black, tortoise or metal finish. To make half-up and ponytails look stylish, and evening or work appropriate.
- Slimline covered elastics to match hair colour, for inconspicuous ponytails.
- Petersham, satin, and velvet ribbon in a variety of colours, in half meter lengths. To cover elastic bands, match an outfit, and add whimsy to a pony.
- Kirby grips/bobby pins. To tame flyaways, wayward fringes and keep up-do's in place.
- Flowers are for the flamboyant but add beautiful country charm on a warm summer's day, they are not for city wear.

Hair accessories pandering to current styles are always found in fast fashion and large retail stores. For a *classic* wardrobe of gorgeous ribbons, source from V.V. Rouleaux or MacCulloch & Wallis. Ribbons look best and less 'girlish' when worn on a low ponytail and with as much *natural* texture kept in the hair as possible. Alice bands and ribbon barettes can be purchased cheaply online, or made at home (the basics purchased at a local haberdashery) with the help of a nimble hand and a glue gun. Fantastic one-off hair flowers and pre-made ribbons on either hair slides or bands can be found on Etsy. Hair elastics, pins, and scrunchies are picked up cheaply at the supermarket or local beauty supply store. Make sure to give them a permanent home in your bathroom or on your vanity and put them to bed every night. It's a horrid feeling wanting to throw your hair up and not a single band or pin can be found. Make a place for them, and re-place them there at the end of every day, else you'll be *replacing* constantly.

Scarves, tippets, wraps, and stoles

It is a general rule that one should match the robustness of her scarf to the fabrics of her outfit, for example tweed and country casuals call for a knitted or woven wool scarf. Lighter dresses call for cottons, and shirting and suiting calls for silks. Formal occasions deserve cashmere wraps or serapes, and perhaps a faux fur tippet if attending a special function. A classic white cotton or linen shirt is elevated with a small silk scarf tied at the neck worn as a necklace. The colour, pattern, and designs of scarves, particularly silk, are a wonderful way to personalise an otherwise plain outfit. Shawls are always useful, perfect for modesty, for extra warmth in winter, and covering bare shoulders in the summertime when the sun briefly (or rudely) hides himself.

Good quality scarves that are designed to last are hard to come by. Fast fashion will fix any temporary bind you may be in to keep out the cold, but for classic and beautiful scarves you'll want to treasure, look to these suppliers:

For art scarves: *English Heritage, The National Gallery, William & Sons.*

For faux fur: *Helen Moore. (Note: real fur just isn't kind, nor a trade an English rose would support).*

For classic neutrals: *Hobbs, Reiss, Brora.*

For casual and country wear: *Joules, Johnstons of Elgin, The House of Bruar, Marks & Spencer.*

For design classics: *Burberry, Lochcarron of Scotland, Joshua Ellis.*

For luxury silks: *Hermes, Liberty London, Beckford Silk, Cordings of Piccadilly, Hawes & Curtis.*

For authenticity: *Hand knitted by your Grandma, or by a maker on Etsy.*

For shawls: *Hawes & Curtis, Cordings of Piccadilly, Lochcarron of Scotland.*

Umbrellas and parasols

Umbrellas are a necessity in British climes, and while a golf umbrella (likely emblazoned with your hairdresser or accounting firm's logo), or cheap folding umbrella from a train station gift shop will suffice in an emergency, you won't know rainfall *luxury* until you invest in a *good* umbrella. For a lady who so often has her hands full with children, handbags, and such things, a mechanical/automatic self-opening umbrella is the most useful kind. You only need to point, press a button, and 'whoosh' your shield is deployed. Automatic umbrellas are generally longer and less totable than a telescopic pocket style which one can stuff into a handbag, but the more robust and well made an umbrella is, the better it will *serve* you. Find preference in a hook handle umbrella where possible so that you can hang it off a crooked arm, or the back of a chair when required. You deserve to buy a good model that you will appreciate for its craftsmanship and strength, and as with anything deemed a style 'investment' you are less likely to lose or forget it when out and about. Cheap umbrellas just aren't cared for. How many times have you walked past a litter bin to see a failed, cheaply produced umbrella stuffed inside it?

A sophisticated umbrella finishes your whole look. There are a surprising variety of colours and designs to choose from to suit anyone's taste. Prices and designs can vary, but a restrained navy or black with mock-horn or wooden crooked handle is a sensible choice and perfect for those working and commuting in town. Royal Warrant holders, Fulton, design a lovely clear birdcage umbrella favoured by the Queen which enables good vision while still offering protection from the rain, they also supply lovely Morris & Co designs, and a rainbow of colours to suit your preference. A personal favourite is the parrot head umbrella sold by James Smith & Sons, perfect for a fan of Mary Poppins. For country life, a large golf umbrella *is* a good idea, but select yours from trusted country brands where testing for these conditions *should* have been considered by the buying team.

Borrow from the boys here too, especially if you are a taller woman, the ladies 'category' only really means they have it in pink. Men's umbrellas tend to be longer and the canopy wider. Considering we are often blessed with horizontal rain, men's umbrellas are far more practical for shielding a friend or a child from the rain, as well as yourself.

Sun Parasols are also a wonderful way to keep the sun off during summer in addition to a hat. You can choose from standard UV parasols that look very similar to normal umbrellas, but for a pretty and very feminine option look at bamboo and paper parasols, or if you'd like to treat yourself to a luxury heirloom consider a Battenberg lace parasol from Pierre Vaux. Bear in mind that lace and paper parasols only provide a little shade and not UV protection (unless otherwise stated). Remember to wear sunscreen.

Umbrella etiquette:

- There's nothing more irritating than being hit in the eye or clobbered in the side of the head with an umbrella. Be aware of those around you and lift your brolly higher than the heads and umbrellas of others when passing on a narrow street or walkway, don't just expect them to walk around you.

- If the person you are passing also has an umbrella, tilt yours to the opposite side, and they *should* do the same to avoid umbrella collision, else if there are people all around and it is impossible or impractical to tilt, the taller person should raise their umbrella over you both.

- Never open an umbrella without first checking the coast is clear around you. Never shake off an umbrella indoors, nor in the proximity of people—

you aren't a soggy dog. Always do it outside and *to* the side, someone might be trying to get in from the rain, don't stand in their way of the door.

- If entering a building, look for an umbrella stand to deposit your brolly or ask for an appropriate place to store where it won't create a puddle on the floor. If one doesn't exist, store it upright (ideally sheltered outdoors), or if inside then out of the way and make sure no one will trip on it.

- Make sure your umbrella is *fully* dry before closing and storing it for any length of time.

- The purchase and application of waterproof 'property of' stickers intended for children's school uniform and equipment is a good way to deter would-be umbrella thieves (they are out there, usually on rainy days). It will clear up any question of to whom the brolly belongs—apply inside the umbrella on the internal frame.

- Lastly, if you are waiting in a queue in the rain and there is a person next to you, whether acquainted to you or not, offer them some shelter, it's only kind. My great grandparents actually met this way; Daisy offered Stanley shelter under her umbrella during a rainstorm in 1930s London—how romantic!

Suppliers: Fulton, London Undercover, Brollies Galore, Aspinal of London, James Smith & Sons, Pasotti, Pierre Vaux, Dubarry, Schöffel.

Belts

For the purpose of holding up one's trousers, and in the case of ladies' fashion, for highlighting the waist. A minimal collection will include a plain black and brown leather (or imitation leather) for the purpose of wearing with trousers or jeans, with the buckle in a metal to suit the individual complexion. Waist cinching belts in lighter tans or whites look lovely to highlight the waist in floaty summer dresses, choose your width to suit the space available at the waist (shorter waists look better with skinnier belts). Elasticated belts can be lovely but be careful they do not fold over themselves. Polo and needlepoint belts match nicely with casual country outfits and summer shorts. A good belt, well chosen and cared for should last for a lifetime, my 'daily' belt worn with jeans is a deep mulberry coloured leather from the 1970s, I have had a few holes punched in over time but it has outlasted every other belt I have bought in a fast fashion store. There are plenty of leather artisans using traditional techniques selling hand crafted belts, many offer personalisation services and emboss initials, making a lovely gift and an investment piece to treasure.

Suppliers: The House of Bruar, The British Belt Company, Pampeano, Crew Clothing, MacKenzie & George, Hicks & Hides, The Cotton London, Tim Hardy.

Gloves

Throughout history and well into the early 1960s it was considered ladylike to wear gloves on *all* occasions outside the home, especially white gloves for daily errands. However with the changing tides it is neither fashionable or expected now. However, the wearing of gloves *can* help keep you from picking up wayward germs and viruses. The Queen mainly wears her gloves in order to keep her health in tip-top condition. Think about the shopping trolleys, keyboards, and door handles you touch throughout the day and what germs they may be harbouring.

Gloves worn during cooler spells need regular laundering, dry cleaning, or at the very least a spritz of disinfectant spray if the fabric isn't too delicate. It is poor form to eat with your gloves on for this very reason, even if you are in the most casual of settings. A lady can choose for herself whether to remove her gloves for shaking hands, (whereas for a man this is quite the opposite—he should always remove his gloves when shaking hands with ladies or other gentlemen). A classic wardrobe of gloves should include:

- Black cotton, fine cashmere, or merino wool, wrist length gloves for formal day wear and funerals.
- Lined leather, suede, or shearling gloves for country wear, in natural leather tones—black, brown, or tan. Some are patched with tweed or tartan which can look very pretty.
- Fine, slim-fit Nappa leather or kidskin in a rainbow of colours for smart work wear and evening wear. Match the tones, colours, and ideally fabrics of your gloves with other accessories.
- Warmer woollen knits, mittens or 'sport' gloves for casual wear in bitter weather and snow.
- Shorties (wrist length) and slightly longer 'gauntlet' gloves are the most versatile lengths and suit most outfits. Elbow length gloves are better suited to evening wear.
- If you want to take a leaf out of the Queen's style book, source her exact white cotton gloves from Cornelia James. Wear with aplomb.

Etiquette & care:

- If you are invited to very formal events, galas, and balls, then opera length gloves are required.
- With regards to jewellery, rings are worn under the glove, while bracelets and dress watches are worn over.

- Remove gloves and place in the lap when dining, or remove and store in a pocket or handbag if dining casually in town.
- If spending leisure time or socialising in a public place then gloves should be removed. It is not necessary to remove them for quick errands at a shop or post office.
- Never fold one glove inside the other (like socks), instead store flat. When out and needing to store in a pocket or handbag, lay one of top of the other and gently fold in half.
- Store flat for long periods.
- If you are wearing gloves with long sleeves, you will want the sleeve to overlap with the hem of your gloves. A flash of bare skin does little to keep you from the cold and also looks a little 'off'—if this look is for fashionable effect, make sure there is enough skin showing to make it look deliberate.

Suppliers: *Dents, Cornelia James, Aspinal of London, William & Sons.*

Shoes

There is something about the mention of a new pair of shoes that sets the heart of many woman aflutter. A beautiful blend of incredible engineering, style, beauty, and craftsmanship that intertwine to birth a gorgeous creature which is also practical! We have to move ourselves about all day and protect our feet from the floor, so why not do so in something we love and consider beautiful?

From woman to woman, I'm the first to admit that it feels hard to adopt a minimalist approach when it comes to shoes, but as we have explored earlier in this book, the strain modern manufacturing practices puts on our earth simply isn't fair. Which is why, instead of encouraging you to pare back on shoes, you should instead be encouraged to become a *connoisseur*. A connoisseur is someone who knows a lot about, and enjoys a particular art form, and as such can judge the levels of quality and skills in that subject. Imagine a beautiful array of footwear options available to you that not only make your heart sing, but are practical, built to last, and make you feel good about yourself (according to how you *carefully considered* the purchase) every time you wear them? How nice does that sound rather than the internal groan that comes when you pull out a pair of cheaply made heels that pinch? Many ladies end up with poor foot health because of substandard quality shoes and this needs to stop! No shoe is worth the pain of bunions, strained arches or tendons, corns, callouses and disfigurement. We pay attention to the careful fitting of our children's shoes, do we not deserve the same level of care? While it is true that if you demand better quality in your accessories you will need to pay a slightly higher price. In the long run, the cost per wear far outweighs the initial investment. Here are some classic footwear styles and manufacturers that create not only pretty shoes for all occasions, but pretty comfortable ones at that.

If you live in the countryside, enjoy walking or own a dog, a trio of country boots, Wellingtons, and walking shoes will likely be the pairs you alternate between frequently, especially if you live in the UK. By nature they have to be on the more robust and tough end of the scale compared to the other shoes in your wardrobe. As such, you need to rely on them for not only protecting your feet from the elements, but being sure they won't let you down on rough terrain or in inclement weather.

Country Boots are ideal for dog walking, equestrian, farming, and outdoor pursuits. They look nice with jeans tucked in, or if kept clean for 'best' with a pair of tights and a country skirt. Country boots are *designed* to be workhorses, they are meant to get muddy and a little bit battered and in most cases, look even better when they do!

Wellington Boots are for the rain. Quite obviously a reason they have been a staple of practical footwear for the English since the early nineteenth century. Ideal for country weekends, dog walking, sporting events, agricultural work, and all manner of menial daily pursuits such as garden maintenance and popping to the shops—these puddle avoiders are most delightful to wear. Pretenders come and go, but a classic 'British Racing Green' pair from Hunter cannot be beaten for staving off 'mizzle', drizzle, and heavy showers. The ladies department offers a rainbow of colours to choose from, and if one wishes even prints. However, 'fashion wellies' won't see you through decades of wear as intended, you'll probably be bored of them after a few seasons. Consider your colour very carefully. Welly liners or shooting socks to line the boot are optional, just make sure to tuck your trousers in to avoid looking silly. Skirts and dresses worn with tights and thick knitwear also look lovely with wellingtons. Just remember, the very point of wearing wellingtons is to avoid getting wet or muddy, *not* to look cool. Store them properly on a rack (upside down) or boot tray to avoid upsetting the carpet, and *always* check for marauding mice and spiders before pulling on a boot—a bitter experience one does not forget in a hurry.

Walking Shoes, Snow & Walking Boots won't always be the most attractive offering in the footwear department, but being caught short in a snowstorm or an impromptu weekend hike will have you appreciating such practical footwear like never before. The fitting of walking shoes and boots is best with a professional in attendance, so these really shouldn't be purchased online in the first instance. Instead head to a specialist outdoor retailer and ask for a fitting, heed their advice with regards to suitable socks and breaking them in. If you are a frequent walker or hiker then you will already know how often your shoes will need replacing, but if you have them for occasional use then they should again, last for many years if well cared for. Walking footwear with good grip is what you want to reach for in Britain's now annual 'big freeze', trainers, wellies, and other boots simply won't do to offer enough protection from slips and falls.

Suppliers: Dubarry, Hunter, Blacks, L.L. Bean, Regatta, Le Chameau, Ariat, The Original Muck Boot Company, Rydale, Toggi, Sorel, Karrimor.

Leather or Suede Riding (or Long) Boots are for smarter days and events, usually worn with country skirts, skinny jeans or moleskins. 'Spanish' style riding boots are icons of country and equestrian style but are easily transferred to town with the wearing of dark jeans and a blazer, or blouse and sweater (especially if they are of black leather). There are many retailers who design and manufacture these boots *in the style of*, to cater to a particular aesthetic, but good quality riding boots, should, with regular care and re-soling, last for many years. There are flat and heeled options, and now many designers offer a way to personalise the look of your boots with inter-changeable coloured zip tassels. Consider also mid-calf cowboy boots in leathers and suedes.

Suppliers: The Spanish Boot Company, Penelope Chilvers, Fairfax & Favor, Russell & Bromley, R. Soles London, The House of Bruar.

Good old Queen Victoria is to thank for making the **Chelsea Boot** fashionable, she clearly liked comfortable footwear and those royals know what's good for them. Designed to be worn and removed with minimal effort, the elastic-sided boot is always popular and as with a gentleman's wardrobe, their streamlined classic looks lend themselves beautifully to both tailored and casual attire. The Chelsea boot is traditionally black leather (and also the most versatile) but incarnations are made in dark brown, and tan leathers, or sueded for country wear. For ladies the Chelsea boot also looks pleasant, cut low on the ankle and worn with skirts and summer dresses.

Suppliers: Clarks, Avesu, Fairfax & Favor, Joseph Cheaney & Sons, Grenson, Chatham, Loake, The House of Bruar.

Court Shoes are the staple shoe for work, parties, and pretty outfits. Their design is classic, refined, and the ultimate in elegance, but not all court shoes are designed, or made equally. The perfect court shoe does not expose the toe cleavage, is of a comfortable mid-height, and the toe an elegant almond shape. The heel is of a width that is sturdy enough to balance your weight, and not so pin-thin you lose it between the cracks in the pavement. Essentially, you want to be able to slip on a court shoe and not notice you are wearing heels at all, which makes finding the best designers so essential. Ideally purchase them from a retailer who *specialises* in shoe design and manufacture, especially if you want your shoes to last. The Court is the one and only shoe that is guaranteed to take you from the office to a party, are thoroughly appropriate for *any* occasion and are timeless enough to pair with almost any outfit from a glitzy dress to denim and a silky evening blouse. One of the leading British designers of court shoes that offer a variety of colours, fabric finishes and heights are L.K. Bennett. Whilst they aren't the cheapest on the market, their price is worth the comfort and the quality, shopping from their permanent range in the sales helps to keep costs low. Year after year their range includes classic courts in a conservative wardrobe of colours, with a few designs made in the 'colour of the season' meaning you can find a court for all occasions. For an attractive price point and comfort, look to Clarks, and Van Dal. Special mention to Hobbs whose designs are classic and also beautifully made.

The key to making your court shoes last is to wipe off any surface dirt before storing in their boxes, kicking off your heels doesn't sound quite as fun when it does damage to your shoes, and ultimately your bank balance. Respect the shoes and they'll respect you. Replace the heel-tips and re-sole annually. There are also plenty of offerings from 'designer' designers too, such as Jimmy Choo, Christian Laboutin, and Valentino who offer court shoes, but as I have never had good reports regarding comfort they do not come approved under the demands for induction into an English rose's permanent wardrobe—unless one has more money than sense. One should not sacrifice the health of her feet, nor spend a working day or evening event in agony, for the sake of her shoes.

Suppliers: *L.K. Bennett, Hobbs, Ferragamo, Gabor, Peter Kaiser, Clarks, Van Dal, Avesu.*

Heeled Sandals for party or occasion wear are something likely bought to 'go with' a particular outfit. They are very pretty offerings but rarely practical, usually only bought and worn once for special evenings or a wedding. If purchased too strappy and too high they will also be unsteady and most uncomfortable—definitely not inspiring to wear again. For this reason we will explore the classics, which, if purchased well and kept in good condition will pair with most new dresses in a wardrobe and therefore negate the need to waste money on shoes that are only destined to clutter up your wardrobe.

A classic suite of heeled sandals include a classic black, a metallic (either gold or silver to suit your complexion), and a light cream or pastel to work with summer outfits. Blacks and metallics work better for evening, whereas a lighter shade may be worn for a daytime event. Consider therefore whether for these occasions you are better placed to invest in a wedge or espadrille which will be more appropriate for summer events which may have you standing on grass or walking on varied terrain. L.K. Bennett offer a nude wedge almond toe court with a braided straw wrap around the heel in their permanent line which will complement most summer outfits.

Suppliers: L.K. Bennett, Rachel Simpson, Charlotte Mills, Hobbs, Van Dal, Kurt Geiger, Stuart Weitzman.

Summer Sandals should have one consideration only, and that is of comfort. Considering how exposed the foot is in a pair of sandals, not to mention how hot one's foot might get, the last thing any woman will want to collect for her feet on a summer's day is a raw blister. Flip-Flops are widely available and incredibly cheap but they offer absolutely no protection or support for the foot, nor elegance. Consider instead a pair of vintage styled Grecian or Spanish 'braided' leather sandals that cover the toes, lower foot, and back of the heel in a caged style offering beauty, ventilation and practicality in one. We tend to be out and about a lot more in summer, whether running errands in town, pottering about the garden, or sightseeing on holiday so the bottom must also have good grip, and the foot bed supportive to the contours of your sole, you *should* be able to walk for miles in them. Really, we should rename flip-flops to flat-foot-flops, it's quite ridiculous how we think they are good enough to be considered 'shoes'. One good pair of tan leather (or imitation) summer sandals that are comfortable and stay on the foot will go with absolutely anything your summer wardrobe can throw at it.

Suppliers: Saltwater Sandals, Pikolinos, Hotter, Clarks, Josef Seibel, Birkenstock, Ecco, Avesu.

Though not traditionally English, sailing days and our rainy streets have made the flat, rubber soled 'good grip' **Moccasin, Driving, Boat/Deck Shoe** a go-to choice for leisure wear for those odd weather days. Namely when it's too cold or drizzly for sandals, but not cold enough for boots or anything more substantial. Easy to slip on, they look great with jeans and chinos in the summer, even dresses. Once you have tried a pair the comfort is unrivalled and will likely have you reaching for trainers less, they look much smarter and in most circumstances are more appropriate than a trainer or sports shoe. They are out of place in a corporate environment but look nicely pulled together for the school run, coffee or lunch with friends, and running errands. Common colours that go with anything are dark brown, and tan. There are lighter and duo-toned pastel or printed offerings for the more adventurous.

Suppliers: Chatham, Rydale, Musto, Orca Bay, Sebago, Dubarry, Tod's.

Trainers or Sports Shoes are worn by the English lady, for exactly that, training or participating in sports. There are a few slimline canvas 'plimsoll' style offerings that can look pretty in a casual setting, but anything more substantial and chunky deserves to be worn with a full sporting outfit. For wearing to the gym, group sports, or an aerobics class, your feet deserve supportive trainers designed for impact and performance. Likewise with walking shoes, your trainers should be properly fitted and 'bought for purpose'. Purchase them in person from a specialist sports store and ask for something suitable according to the sport you will be performing. Running for example requires a slimline trainer with forward flexibility, whereas a trainer worn for tennis needs side impact moulding. Forget fashion and buy something that will look after your feet.

Suppliers of pretty plimsolls: Veja, Superga, Keds, Converse, Vans.
Suppliers of performance trainers: New Balance, Nike, Adidas, Asics.

A ladies **Penny Loafer or Brogue/Oxford Shoe** is a smart form of a slip-on. Often styled in patent or calf-leather with a penny-slip, snaffle, or bit across the top of the foot (in the case of loafers), and laces for Oxford and brogues they make a formal alternative to a casual shoe on occasions where you might not want to, or it is deemed impractical to wear heels. These flat but smart shoes work well with tailoring and skirts for work wear and are a good shoe for daughters at school. Tan or brown leather or suede work well for casual outfits and country wear.

Suppliers: The House of Bruar, Clarks, G.H. Bass & Co.

Of course there are many other styles of shoes and options available to us all, but the suggestions given are those that have made the grade for not only complementing a British lifestyle and our climate, but their versatility, practicality, and promotion of good foot health.

A guide to shoe buying, wearing, and etiquette:

- Buy shoes well in advance of any event you may require them for. They all need a period of 'breaking in' for maximum comfort.

- If they feel uncomfortable in any way in the store, they won't feel any better at home. Put them back on the shelf.
- Heels should not make you feel as though you will topple forwards or backwards, if that is the case they are not the right height for your frame.
- Toes should never extend beyond the toe-bed of a shoe. Either they are too small, or the straps too loose and the shoe is unsupportive. Avoid!
- Just because they are trendy or fashionable doesn't mean you should own or covet them.
- To quickly break in a pair of slightly too tight shoes; wear with thick socks and heat with a hairdryer (on the foot) then allow the shoe to cool completely while still on the foot.
- Remove ALL stickers from the sole of a shoe before wearing in public.
- If toes or heels are exposed, keep them nicely manicured and moisturised.
- Remove your shoes if your host asks you to.
- Remove shoes when entering your own home to avoid traipsing dirt onto carpets and rugs.
- Do 'the twist' on gravel to add grip to a new sole.

It is worth investing in:

- **Shoe Trees.** To keep the shape of your shoes. Available in plastic and coated in flock, but far nicer and planet friendly options are available in cedar wood, which are a little pricier but also help to deodorise.
- **Valet Box.** Invest in a specialist kit which includes all polish, creams, brushes, and cloths to keep shoes and leather goods clean and nourished, invaluable for the longevity of handbags especially!
- **Shoe Bags.** If your shoes didn't come with them, buy in brushed cotton to protect shoes and surrounding items from scratches and dirt when packing for travel.

Handbags and purses

Alongside shoes, there is no greater addition to the wardrobe that can offer an instant update or change of look to an outfit than a handbag. There are too many options available to explore every style, and therefore we will refine our choices to the backbone of a capsule handbag collection that will provide you with something appropriate and practical for all occasions. The price points of bags can vary greatly but most women are highly attuned to a particular 'model' of bag that they like and are happy to spend their money on. Do make sure however that you invest in something that will last you for as long as possible. Handbags really are workhorses, and your investment should reflect that in quality and longevity.

The **Cross-Body Bag** is indispensable for busy ladies, and especially those who are a little 'forgetful'. Not only that, they are the handbag least likely to get snatched from you in busy scenarios. A good cross body bag will have an adjustable strap long enough to sit across your frame with enough 'slack' for you to be able to reach into the bag while you are still wearing it. My favourite kind is a light, soft and flexible leather (or leather like material), in a medium size; enough for a purse, notebook, phone, glasses case, and keys (plus room to spare) with a few internal pockets for lipstick, powder, a small hairbrush, and tissues. It must not be adorned with 'embellishments' or non-functioning metal attachments. Even though the weight is distributed across the body, unnecessary weight caused by decoration can soon feel rather heavy and wasteful. It also must have a zip, for privacy and security. Take your cross body bag when shopping, as leaving a handbag in a trolley is not sensible (I learned this the hard way). They are also the bag of choice for days out where you might be walking for long periods of time—toting a bag in your hands is tiring and not enjoyable.

The **Tote Bag** is a big old sack capable of filling until it busts at the seams. Sadly Mary Poppins' bag hasn't been invented yet and this is the closest we have come and they are attractive to new mothers and ladies who use public transport to commute to work. Be mindful of how inelegant and disorganised a stuffed-to-the-brim bag can look in formal or work settings, so clear it out as often as you can. If you do like a roomy tote bag, then consider buying a few 'inner organisers' such as canvas pouches to group together belongings into categories, you can pull out what you need as and when rather than having to dig for treasure every time you need a pen or a breath mint. Tote bags are also magnets for boyfriends and friends who cannot be bothered to carry their own items, you'll quickly realise that a smaller bag means you aren't treated like a pack horse.

The **Clutch or Evening Bag** is a place to invest your money (wisely) if you are a real lover of handbags. The infrequency of use (to protect it from daily knocks) and pleasure you'll get when taking out such a beautiful item will increase the feeling of excitement surrounding the event. I know a handbag is only a 'thing', but to have that one special item in your wardrobe you have long saved for and treat like a pet is what true luxury feels like. You only need one. One classic piece, in a classic colour, in a classic design with absolutely no fashionable or *of the moment* embellishments. Buy with consideration and conservatism and that one handbag will go with everything. Think about buying a secondhand piece, let some other lady take the hit on the depreciation of such a classic.

The **Top Handle Handbag** is a smart choice for the lady who works in a corporate environment, or a pretty and more formal option for nice days out, it isn't as secure as a cross body bag but works better where you might not want the line of your outfit interrupted or wrinkled. Some top handle bags come with a detachable long handle to enable you to carry it over one shoulder. Be aware that this offers you less freedom of movement as well as security. Avoid the 'lean' to counterbalance too much weight if you are overloaded. As with any handbag, keep the internal contents as pared down as possible. You shouldn't have to dig around for more than a few seconds to find what you are looking for, nor carry any weight that is more than necessary. Many ladies like to buy their handbags in their 'signature colour', which is a fabulous idea if that colour will tone with the rest of your wardrobe. Otherwise, look for a neutral colour such as black, navy, tan, dark brown, or a deep maroon. Remember that the more print or detailing a bag has, the quicker it will date. Match neutral coloured bags to outfits by wrapping a silk scarf around the handles. There are many tutorials online demonstrating how to do this. If you want a bag to last you a long time, then look for something with good solid structure. Care for your bags as much as you do your shoes and they will serve you for a long time.

The **Purse or Wallet** is as important to keep clear of clutter as any handbag. Choose a style that has enough room for a little cash, some coins, and your debit cards, plus space to stuff a receipt or two. For all store cards (membership, not credit) download a mobile app that will reproduce the barcode for you for easy scanning. Not only does it reduce the clutter in your purse, should you misplace it, or your purse gets stolen, it negates the need to request copies of all that plastic—a whole lot of administration you don't need in a time of stress. Your purse will also pick up lots of germs. If material allows, clean it regularly with anti-bacterial wipes and a disinfectant spray.

Suppliers: Modalu, Mulberry, Radley, Aspinal of London, Osprey London, Chanel, L.K. Bennett, Launer London, Vendula London, Yoshi, Ladbante London, Matt & Nat, J.W. Pei, The Cambridge Satchel Co.

Loungewear and pyjamas

Do you remember when we discussed how you set the tone for your home? Also how what one wears will reflect how one feels about oneself? What you wear around the house in the dead of night and during those quiet evenings deserves as much attention and respect as your daily wardrobe. Your bedtime style should consist of more than paint-splattered oversized t-shirts and ripped leggings. Comfortable they may be, there's no denying that, but attractive they are not.

There are plenty of gorgeous **Nightdresses** available to suit the coldest of winter nights to balmy summer evenings. White cotton is a classic look, and Victorian inspired nightdresses are whimsical and appropriate. Always consider whether a nightdress is too short, low cut, or thin. If you wouldn't be happy to answer the door in it during an emergency, or walk around wearing it in company then it's probably not suitable. The same goes for your **Pyjamas**, classic button-down styles in a material thick enough to keep you modestly covered will mean you can enjoy your breakfast with the in-laws at leisure on Christmas morning instead of being red-faced. You also just *cannot* beat the comfort of flannel pyjamas in the winter! Invest also in a nice **Dressing Gown or Robe**. Towelling robes are nice for wearing after a shower, but a tailored cotton, waffle, or velvet robe is nicer for company and for unexpected stays in hospital. They are also useful to take when travelling, a dash to reception or the shared loo in the dead of night deserves a little coverage and comfort on your part. If you want all-out luxury then silk anything for nighttime is a statement and something to treasure.

Suppliers: *David Neiper, Bonsoir of London, Marks & Spencer, The White Company, The 1 for U, P.J. Pan, Olivia Von Halle.*

Slippers

Classic and classy slippers for wearing round the house are surprisingly hard to find. Ideally, in order to get the best life out of your slippers, look for something with a semi-sturdy sole rather than a self-fabric sole. Whether your slippers are slip-on 'scuff' style, or encase the entire foot is dependent on what you are comfortable wearing around the house. They are not only designed to keep the feet warm, but you should consider them your 'indoor shoes', which means you can and *should* remove your outdoor shoes as soon as you enter the house to avoid traipsing in dirt. Just as you should never wear your outdoor shoes inside, do not wear your slippers outside for even the briefest of moments—grabbing the washing in or running something to the bin counts too. For this reason, garden shoes akin to 'Crocs', Birkenstocks, or clogs are ideal for leaving by the back door if you just need to pop out, and which is why I personally prefer a 'scuff' style slipper which are easier to slip on and kick off in haste. There are also really pretty boudoir style slippers, as well as velvet smoking slippers available, but pick according to your lifestyle. As lovely as it may be having a pair of white marabou mules for around the house, they'll begin to look rather tired very quickly if you wear them while doing the housework.

Suppliers: Moorlands Sheepskin, David Neiper, Uggs, Birkenstock, Celtic & Co.

Underwear and undergarments

Ladies, you do *not* have to wear a bra. In case you didn't know, it is *not* a legal requirement for a woman to encase her breasts in a contraption designed to constrict and compress one of the most natural parts of her body for the sake of societal pressure and expectation. Where we are of course going to advise *for* the case of being publicly decent and a little bit modest, wearing a device that digs-in and makes you feel uncomfortable is not the only way to achieve this. Nipples are not taboo either, and if you feel comfortable enough without all the cantilevered and highly engineered 'support', a soft bralette for a little support, extra warmth and modesty may be all you need, especially if you are small breasted. Ladies with an ample bosom who like the support a bra offers absolutely must see a specialist fitter to ensure that she is wearing the correct size. Remember that your size is not universal across all manufacturers and you may need to have a fitting in several stores, or for several ranges if purchasing from a department store. Never rush when looking for new lingerie or 'blind buy' a bra if you have the opportunity to try it on first. If shopping from home make your order with the idea in mind that you *may* need to send it back to the retailer if the fit is not suitable. Check if they offer free returns (or accept returns at all).

If you have a wardrobe of classic, modest pieces it is likely you will not need an all-singing all dancing bra that allows for the straps to be removed, crossed over, or slung about the neck and 'padded' to the high heavens. Nor do you need a bra bedecked in diamantes and unnecessary embellishments. These 'fashion' bras are generally sold to appeal to women who favour plunging necklines and clothing that exposes too much skin and breast to be tasteful. If you have a gown for an event that does not work with a particular bra in your collection already, then shop for a new bra and take the dress along with you to ensure it works.

The exposure of a bra strap is not the end of the world, but do make sure you aren't exposing more than you should in the name of 'fashion'. This is also the case for the visibility of a bra underneath a shirt—it may be sexy, but is it appropriate? Is it distracting for others, particularly in the workplace or in family environments?

Bras should be replaced yearly at least, and ideally hand washed after every couple of wears. Special nets can be purchased at a reasonable cost to protect both the delicate construction of your underwear and the other clothes you wash them with from snags that may be caused by the hooks or underwire of the bra itself. Re-shape the cups of the bra after washing and hang to air dry to increase longevity. Tumble driers will murder all sense of shaping and elastication.

If you find a bra that fits well and makes you feel good, invest in as many as you can afford. It's easy to fall in love with a 'favourite' bra, but it is not ladylike, nor good for your health to wear it to death. Worse still when you go to re-purchase and find they don't make that model anymore. Having a few means they will get equal wear and you can enjoy the design for longer.

Buy your bras from specialist manufacturers, fast fashion stores offer them cheaper of course but they are far from superior. Remember, comfort trumps price *and* 'fun' designs. Your bras are worn *under* things for a reason, pay no more heed to them than for their comfort and cleanliness. If you want *sexy* underwear buy it for those occasions where you get to enjoy the novelty of it, but do not rely on it daily. Your bra should serve you, and you are not a slave to it just because you are told that's just the way things are.

Comfort for the girls first, girls!

Suppliers: *Triumph, Rigby & Peller, Wacoal, Miss Mary, Royce, Sloggi, Gossard, Marks & Spencer.*

Knickers

The advice for knickers is exactly the same for the covering of the breasts. Wear what it comfortable for *you*, not what you are told is sexy or what you feel is expected of you. If larger full brief 'granny' knickers are your thing then good for you! They are the most comfortable, healthy, and versatile option out there! Where you think they might be visible under your clothing they are actually the most discreet as the waistband sits directly under the waistband of your clothing, and the pant-line under the crease of your bottom. It's better to expose a bottom clad in cotton than a bare cheek when the wind whips up your skirt too! Think of Marilyn, not a thong in sight for that girl. In the golden age and pin-up era, all those classic beauties had larger knickers. In many things, less is more, but not when it comes to your pants!

Wearing underwear that is too tight and sits too close to your undercarriage actually increases the risk of infection, plus all kinds of hot and uncomfortable situations 'down there'. Natural fibres with a gusset that protects for modesty and space enough for the comfortable use of sanitary products is the ideal scenario. Thongs and g-strings have had their time in the sun but are not suitable *daily* underwear for the sake of your health. Multi-packs of knickers in

100% cotton can be bought for a very reasonable price at most supermarkets and departments stores and are probably the only thing that slips through the net of the "buy to last" mindset. Underwear needs frequent washing and replacing so buy with abandon and repurchase as soon as they begin to lose their elastic or look tired and faded.

For pretty knickers, 'occasion' knickers, and performance underwear that shows no seams etc look to the brands that manufacture your bras. They often offer matching designs in a shape to suit your bottom half preferences, whether a full brief, thong, or boy short.

Suppliers: Triumph, Rigby & Peller, Sloggi, Marks & Spencer, Organic Basics, Rossell England, or your local supermarket.

Socks, stockings, and tights

Everyone needs socks, make sure yours are 100% cotton or made of as much natural fibre in the composition as possible so that your feet can breathe and will not retain dampness. Otherwise you risk obtaining bacterial infections in the foot. Synthetic socks also make the foot smell. Wash your socks after *every* wear for good hygiene.

Knee-highs and tights are very useful for an extra layer of warmth under trousers and jeans in the winter, and of course for the wearing with skirts and boots or brogues in the cooler months. There are plenty of deniers and colours to choose from and can be a useful tool to tie the colours of an outfit together. For winter, dark grey can be a softer and more flattering option for casual wear than black. Ribbed tights are also beautiful for styling with country outfits.

It is good etiquette to wear sheer tights for formal events, and is a rule observed by the ladies of the royal households. Some corporate environments call for this too. They provide a smoother even look for the skin on the legs, and provide modesty with lighter dresses for day events or formal dresses in the evening.

If you are wearing an open toed shoe, you will need to purchase special open-toed sheer tights, or go without. If you feel you need it, a smooth and even tone for the skin on your legs can be achieved with a little foundation make up mixed with a drop of moisturiser, and then set with a dusting of translucent powder. Avoid being too heavy handed, it will look obvious and could be at risk of 'transferring'—less is more.

- If you wear tights frequently, it pays to purchase a pair of white cotton gloves for the putting on of your tights. It will mean you are less likely to snag the delicate knit with a nail or piece of jewellery.
- Wash your tights in a net bag to avoid tangles and unnecessary 'pulling'.
- Carry an extra pair of tights with you in your bag for an event, or keep a pair in your desk drawer for immediate replacement if you get a snag or a ladder.
- Holes, snags and ladders can never be repaired. Retire tired tights and socks as soon as they show wear.
- Avoid drying socks and tights in the tumble drier.
- If you have a larger foot, consider shopping the men's section for socks as they will likely shrink with washing.
- Pair socks inside one another for easy finding, fold tights loosely, and store together in a cotton drawstring bag. Storing them loose with other items invites stretching, tangles, and damage.

Suppliers: The Sock Shop, Thought Clothing, Green Fibres, Wolford, Pretty Polly, Aristoc, Falke.

Camisoles & Slips are fantastic tools for making sheer blouses and dresses feel a little more modest, and can offer an extra layer for warmth and comfort in almost all circumstances. A full slip can work with a dress or separates (not trousers), while a blouse and skirt will need separate vests or half slips. Choose yours in a nude for versatility, and check that the material is made from a non-static material. It is best to wear them slightly larger for comfort. A restrictive slip never feels good and can get incredibly hot. It is surprising how feminine one can feel wearing a slip too! In the depths of winter, consider investing in some **Thermal Underwear** separates in cotton, wool, or bamboo to layer under your clothing. They help to retain heat but also offer the chance to wear things that would otherwise be 'out of season' if their material is a little thin to wear alone. Thermals can be purchased as vests, short and long sleeved tops, as well as in long 'shorts' for wearing under tights and skirts or indeed trousers.

Suppliers: David Neiper, Marks & Spencer, Patra, British Thermals.

The responsibility and care taking of a wardrobe

Now you have greatly considered the purchasing of new items for your wardrobe that you intend to last for many years and remain looking their tip top best, it is a good idea to get to grips with proper housekeeping and optimum care for your items. With most of us belonging to a 'throw it in the

For the washing of our bodies with **Soap** in the bath or shower, for too long we have been convinced by cosmetics companies that we need harsh detergents, perfumes, and suds to get really clean. In fact, nature intended for us to use *just* water, and in all cases this is true. Consider switching to a natural, organic soap made from plant derived ingredients if you like the feeling of soap and the perfume it leaves. Package free soaps are making a comeback and can easily be picked up in your local health food store. They last longer and are more environmentally friendly than all those plastic bottles on your bathroom shelf. The scents are wonderful and natural compared to those made with synthetic fragrances. Explore beautiful classic English soap manufacturers if the natural route isn't your thing.

Suppliers: Conchus Life, Wild Sage & Co, Faith in Nature, Little Soap Company, Floris London, Woods of Windsor, Bronnley England.

The scent or **Perfumes** a lady uses are likely to be ones that she is already in love with. Many women have a signature scent or two that they use for day and night wear, something that is nostalgic to them and evokes certain memories. Your olfactory senses can give so much pleasure and remember so many unique things according to scent. A few alternative perfumes may creep into your collection for very hot, or cold weather as some light or heavier scents suit different climates and seasons. What works for you in damp midwinter England may not be quite so lovely in Tuscany. Select your perfume according to your lifestyle, personal taste and what works for *you*, rather than deferring to the latest trends and what is fashionable at the moment. The scent you choose *must* make a tasteful and good impression. Do not douse yourself so much so that it swallows you whole. A simple spritz on a few pulse points is enough. The aim is to enhance, not overpower. All perfumes finish and 'dry down' differently on everyone according to their individual skin chemistry. In order to find out what works for you is all a case of trial and error.

There are a handful of heritage English perfume houses who know how to select a unique scent to complement your tastes. They explain the compositions of perfumes very well so that you can get a feel for the perfume as a whole, not just its trendy name or trusting it based on celebrity endorsement. Always buy samples to test the chemistry against your body and whether they work with your personal style before investing in full bottles. Trial the scent for at least a week before committing. Mainstream brands sometimes offer smaller vials, though you will have better luck purchasing samples from heritage perfumers.

Suppliers: Atkinson's of London, Bronnley England, Floris London, Joe Malone, Miller Harris, Molton Brown, Penhaligon's, Yardley.

Hair

The cut and style you choose for your hair is as personal to you as your DNA and everyone has the right to embrace what is right for her. Yet for the sake of your hair health, do avoid putting it through the mill for the sake of trends. If you want a classic English rose look, then consider a cut that is as fuss-free as possible and allows you to wash, dry, brush, and go. Too many hours are spent taming and wrestling with our strands in order to fit into an *ideal* of what beautiful hair is. When in actual fact, the most beautiful hair you can have for yourself is embracing the natural colour and texture you were born with. If you care for your hair with natural shampoos with *good* ingredients, keep it well moisturised, free of harsh chemicals such as bleach, dye and styling products *and* avoid heat at all costs then your crowning glory will reward you in no time. For hair that refuses to grow, consider shunning all heat and chemical processes and concentrate on improving your diet. Our genetics play a role in the natural maximum length our hair can achieve, but there is always something you can do to help it along a little if that's what you wish. Good tools are also essential for the care of your hair, so invest in brushes and tools that are manufactured to the highest standards. A comb from the pound shop will *not* do if you want a beautiful mane.

Regardless of hair colour and type, take good care of it. A neat cut and a good brushing are all you need to look neat and presentable. Opting for a ponytail is helpful on those days where you feel your hair won't behave.

For formal hairstyles, the proper look for an English rose is always a little 'undone'. That does not mean she is unkempt, but instead there is a looseness and softness in a formal style for evenings, galas and weddings. Take inspiration from the Duchess of Cambridge for modern formal hairstyling done the right way.

Suppliers of brushes and combs: Kent Brushes, Mason Pearson.

Suppliers for cleansing: Aveda, Faith in Nature, Rahua, Wild Sage & Co, Conchus Life, John Masters Organics, Jason, Natura Siberica.

Nails on both the hands and feet should be kept meticulously clean, short, and well-groomed for daily life and work. English ladies are not ones to wear avant-garde nail designs with embellishments or crazy colours. Stick with pale buff nudes, natural pinks, or soft corals. For evenings and events a nude, or for adventure, a classic red is the best option. Long nails are of course pretty (in most cases) but also pretty impractical. Take care if you wish to wear colour (whether simple polish or professional gel) on your nails that you give the nail bed opportunity to breathe from time to time. Investment in a good nail clipper, nail brush for beside the sink, and nail file are essential. A buffer is also a nice addition if you have the time and enjoy a bit of DIY. If you are not confident in the grooming of your cuticles, a simple 'shape' and spruce up (ask for no polish) at a beauty salon will only set you back a couple of pounds and ten minutes. At the very least, don't forget to moisturise your hands and feet, especially around the nails with a good emollient, or a bit of coconut oil before bed will do!

If you are a nail biter, invest in some clear 'stop biting' nail polish readily available online, and wear white cotton gloves to bed. In some cases the application of artificial acrylic nails or a gel polish can help break the cycle of nail biting, but they aren't the best option for long term health of the nail.

Suppliers of tools: Boots, supermarkets, or beauty supply stores.
Suppliers of polish: Revlon, Essie, Nails Inc London.

The very idea of **Make Up** is to *enhance* the beauty you already have, not to mask it or create something that isn't there at all. All this modern contouring, shaping and blending puts so many young ladies in front of the mirror for the hours they should be out enjoying the sunshine, reading a good book, or spending time with their friends and loved ones. This obsession with a made up face can only add to feelings of inadequacy and moves us further away from the celebration of natural beauty. It is most definitely not aligned to classic English values.

An English rose will wear a foundation or dusting of powder that simply offers a little coverage and evening out of skin tone. Then masking discolouration with a concealer, only when and where she needs it. A light shaping and filling in of the eyebrow's natural shape in a colour to match the hair there (no drawing overly exaggerated shapes with a sharpie). A little blush in a natural colour on the apples of her cheeks, a light eyeshadow to brighten up the lid and to mask any blue or red veins on the eyelid. Perhaps a line of pencil or powder eyeliner at the lash line in a dark brown or grey. Then a swipe of mascara to define the lashes. Any bronzing is performed by kisses from the sun.

Her greatest extravagance is a lipstick which she chooses in a shade to flatter her skin-tone and the natural colour of her tooth enamel.

There are countless 'natural' makeup brands now springing up in the beauty market. Where once the witchcraft of how these lotions and creams were made was hidden from us, ladies the world over are demanding to know where, how, and at whose cost their cosmetics are made. Avoid makeup manufactured in China at all costs, these products are often found as cheap 'gift sets' in pharmacy stores. Instead invest your money in make up that acts like skincare, contains better (organic) ingredients, and where possible, is guaranteed cruelty free.

Suppliers: Dr. Hauscka, Inika Beauty, W3ll People, RMS Beauty, Ere Perez.

For beautiful eyes, look for the good in others; for beautiful lips, speak only words of kindness; and for poise, walk with the knowledge that you are never alone.

Audrey Hepburn

What to wear where

There are plenty of 'etiquette' rules on what should be worn to each and every occasion. Frankly, many of them are hard to keep up with and largely outdated, but if you would like a quick summary of what a true Englishman or Englishwoman would *remember* in order to make quick sartorial decisions rather than hunt them out in a specific text book, this list of key pointers is all you need:

- If in doubt dress up, it brings about a sense of occasion and 'joy of the moment'.
- For weddings, *never* wear white.
- For interviews, keep it modest and incredibly neat. Let your *personality* do the talking.
- For dates, keep it attractive and modest. If you wouldn't meet their parents in it, think again.
- Religious buildings: Ladies: Knees covered, shoulders covered, ideally no open toed shoes (hair covered if requested). Men: jacket on, shirt tucked-in and ties on.
- For formal events, take your cue from a British royal closest to you in age.

CONCLUSION

THE BASICS OF THE ENGLISH LIFESTYLE

The art of living an English lifestyle, given to you in a nutshell

We won't argue the fact that it is rather important to make a good impression in how you present yourself and display your manners. All etiquette books that have gone before concentrate so hard on 'the done thing' concerning cutlery placement, how to pen a thank you note, what to wear, and the order of precedence at a top table, but in no way is this helpful to the masses. I for one have never dined with royals, nor am I likely to so. Is it not more realistic to concentrate our efforts on *daily* manners and getting ourselves into a frame of mind that makes common life a little more amiable?

After all these chapters I do hope you have realised by now that it is the attitude towards others that you keep in your heart and what comes *out of your mouth* that are the most important elements of all. You don't have to speak in a posh voice or use fancy language in order to be considered a person of refinement and good manners. You just need to *have* good manners, and know deep in your heart what those things are!

Many of us carry other people's words in our hearts, allowing them to affect our daily lives, and some of those things may have been spoken to us when we were very young. Words have the power to shape, influence, and harm us. Words can change levels of self-esteem, inspire us to withdraw or communicate, despise or love other people. Words, according to which ones you *choose* can be both equally uplifting or debilitating. Sometimes speaking hard truths is essential but even so it *must* be done out of love.

This is why, what you say *to* people says more about **you** than it does about *them*. If we spoke only words of kindness, gentleness, and grace then it would go some way (in fact, probably a significant way) to creating a happier nation of people.

Cast your mind on the wealth of globally exported period dramas such as Austen, Downton Abbey, Victoria, The Crown… now think of the way the protagonist characters speak to each other so politely and eloquently. *This* is the charm that makes the English lifestyle so appealing to people the world over. It lies in our inherent respect for one another, our care-taking of our neighbour before ourselves, and using *graceful* language to express this level of respect and consideration. That is what gives this English nation our reputation for good manners and gentility. Believe it or not, posh accents are *not* the main ingredient for being truly English. Kind and considerate words are. There are small pockets of society and individuals living within this nation that lead their lives according to these quiet traditions, modesty, and good morals. Living a genteel English lifestyle is *a choice one makes for oneself*, **regardless** of where you might live.

You can be the most handsome man, or the prettiest girl in the world but unless you speak and draw your actions from a place of kindness, then outward beauty or riches can only take you so far.

We must learn to think before we speak *and* act. Now so used to living in a society of immediacy, our learned impatience has influenced our communication too. We used to be happy to wait for a snail-mail reply with carefully crafted and considered words, yet we now sling text messages and emails back and forth with abandon. Our mouths have begun to sling words around too without much regard for the outcome. It really is a good thing to keep your mouth shut if you don't have anything nice to say, doing so reflects rather poorly on you.

The English choose to craft their conversation to reflect their emotional intelligence rather than just dish out 'empty talk'. Empty talk is when a person goes on and on about things that in the grand scheme of things won't make a *difference* to the subject being discussed. Many people talk just to be heard and to be the centre of attention, yet don't have anything to add to the conversation, or create any richness. This doesn't mean to say that you should only speak when there is a solution, but don't chat mindlessly to fill the void or to be heard.

One of the easiest ways in which to show someone you care about them is to sit back, shut up, and listen, not talk over them! Asking leading questions will bring richness to a conversation. To show that you are listening, respond with encouraging statements and questions but leave out the selfish sentences. Be kind, even when you may disagree. In many social group conversations and definitely in private ones, people are communicating with you in order to *hear and feel* your acceptance and encouragement, not judgement and condemnation. People love nothing more than to talk about themselves. English ladies and gentlemen are careful not to fall into the trap of making every single conversation about them, demonstrating they care what others have to say.

Be quick to listen and slow to speak

In his book 'How to Win Friends and Influence People', Dale Carnegie makes a valid point that those who win friends easily are those who truly listen, always speak kindly of others, are very slow to speak, and are very considered in what they say. This, dear friends is the central *value* and motivation behind good etiquette.

People like to talk about themselves. Some people manage the balance of conversation well, giving equal air time to both the listener and what they have to say, but the worst conversationalists are those who constantly harp on about themselves. You know the type, nothing is more important than their opinion, what they are doing, and all the minute details about their lives. Often these people do not filter what they share and often find themselves regretting the information they spill.

Be sure to carefully think about the balance of conversations you have, do you speak too much about yourself and your opinions? Are you giving your friend room to speak? Being quick to listen and slow to speak not only shows that you are interested in what others have to say, but it also helps you to guard your heart and keep a little mystery. *Wait* for people to ask you for your opinion on something they might have said, sometimes an interjected opinion is most unwelcome. Not everyone cares what you think about *everything*. Of course, if you are in an intimate setting whereby the conversation is taking on a debate/advice-giving tone then your opinions and interjections might be welcome, but in most situations, particularly when you don't know someone well, your opinions could land you in hot water. Opinions sometimes hurt other parties when delivered blindly.

Encourage, encourage, encourage

There is nothing better you can do for other people than to *encourage* them. We are sadly lacking an encouraging culture, instead we choose to look for the negative in a situation, or we like to take a competitive edge and it pains us to pay someone a compliment or encourage them when they are doing well.

Positive encouragement is a true sign of love and compassion for people. We encourage our children when they are doing well, as do we with people who are most dear to us, but why do we stop there? Do you not love to hear compliments and praise when you accomplish something good? Words contain so much positive power when they are delivered with encouragement, love, and enthusiasm. You should be dishing it out like it is going out of fashion. If you are proud of someone, impressed by something they have achieved, or think in your mind a compliment about them then share it! Share it out loud, or communicate it in any way that is appropriate. This is where social media can be used for great things. Share a status of something good you might be feeling about your friend, loved one, or even someone in the public eye who is doing something you admire, rather than using it to complain or berate. Encouragement and love is the very definition of what makes a kind person. It is the very essence of what sets us apart from the animal kingdom.

Would you not like to be complimented and encouraged by those around you? It's what makes our society great, so *trade in encouragement.*

Help, help, help

Words are powerful, we know this, and I have done nothing but force feed you this message throughout these pages, but what works greater than any word at certain times is **action**.

Sometimes you have to muck in and help. Get your hands dirty and your life and energy engaged with someone else's 'issue' or whatever they have to deal with. This can range from helping out when someone is sick, helping to take care of their pet when they go away, making meals for a new family when a baby arrives, or passing on the details of a great lawyer when the proverbial hits the fan.

We like to kid ourselves that we are always busy, that giving a few pounds a month to a charity is 'enough', but what people need isn't your excuses or reluctant help, they need your time and your compassion. People all around you need your help.

In every situation when you hear there is difficulty, or someone's circumstances are changing for the best or worst, always think about what you can do to help. What do you have that you can share? It may not be much in terms of material offerings, but your sacrificed time is invaluable. An offer to babysit, a lift to work for a colleague whose car is in for servicing. Picking up groceries for someone with an illness. Spending time with an old friend who is suffering with loneliness after a bereavement. Think about people and their circumstances *beyond* what they show you. Consider your elderly neighbour when a snow storm hits—are they warm enough, do they have milk in the house? Your friend whose washing machine has broken down that she can't afford to replace, perhaps you can't afford to fix it for her, but you *can* do a load or two of washing. Just think, "What action can I take that might make someone's day that little bit easier?" You'll want people to think of *you* when you find yourself in a sticky situation. Be reliable, amiable, and willing to give your time. You never know when you might need the time and assistance from someone yourself. The odds are, you are more likely to get back what you give out. People remember those who help them in times of need, both great and small. This is called 'applied human**kind**.' Be the help and give the gift of time.

Stop chasing happiness

Finding happiness is something we all strive for, but also one of the toughest things to do and achieve. Quite often we feel like the world is conspiring against our happiness. Jobs are lost, holidays cancelled, relationships sour, we find we can't afford a bigger home or the latest tech. Happiness, my darling, is somewhat of an illusion, have you ever met anyone that was truly happy? If you've come across someone you would consider to be happy or claim they are, it's likely they are living rather simply, and I'll bet they have a countenance of peace, contribution, and kindness about them.

Think about that—we are constantly sold the idea of what we can do, or buy, to reach or implement a state of happiness. You must buy 'this thing', or 'go here' and it'll make you happy. From holidays, to relationships, diet pills, a bigger home, a new car, the list goes on and on. These things are replaced season after season so you find yourself upgrading, or saving for *more*. So we stop sharing time and resources with others because we are always trying to *get* more things for *ourselves*.

Life is a journey, and not all journeys are smooth, there will be bumps in the road. The measure of the Englishman is how he copes and what he does in those seasons. He will pull his socks up and do something to change whatever it is that is causing him discomfort. It's how we won the war. We kept calm and got on with it.

Action brings about change, and change means that a situation will move from one state to another. This goes for any challenge, real or emotional.

Instead of aiming for, or trying to *buy* happiness, an achievable goal is to aim for *contentment* instead. You can be content with very little! Imagine the sense of relief you'll feel when you begin to chase experiences and enriching relationships rather than status and possessions. Imagine how much more exciting your life would be spent building relationships and contributing to the world, even with a smile and a cheery hello to a stranger in the morning.

Contentment and learning to be happy with what you already have, the things you have already achieved, the power and potential you have *within* you to change things, and the opportunity you have to change your life *will* make you feel better.

Caring for others, and being deliberately kind to those around you brings an enormous sense of wellbeing. Life lived outside of your own head and emotions is really rather pleasing, it brings purpose to our lives.

Don't seek happiness, seek quiet contentment. When we look too far in the distance for our utopia we lose sight of the wonderful things right under our own nose. If we just cross our eyes and 'lose focus' and not worry about what the outside world *says* will make you happy, you may just discover you already have it.

Faster and newer is not better, busy is not more important. What you *think* is important really isn't when your life and the wellbeing of those around you is under threat.

If you want to know the true art of etiquette, it is not held in social position, or a table setting. It is the position of your heart.
Alena Kate Pettitt

Lastly, and this is the most important lesson of ALL

If there is one word that expresses all the lessons in this book, and one to take away with you in order to embrace and live this English lifestyle, it is … 'consideration'.

Hold this word in your heart and think of it before you leap.

• Consider what you are about to say *before* you say it. Empty talk holds no value. Harmful talk is never forgotten.
• Consider what you'll do with your time and whether it is enriching before you spend it. You won't get it back.
• Consider what you read and what you watch, is it good for you, affirming, inspiring, uplifting?
• Consider how you are occupying a space physically, are you being considerate towards those around you?

- Consider what you buy before you buy it, do you need it, can you afford it, do you want to purchase it to fill a void?
- Consider what you are eating, or feeding your children, is it healthy, wholesome and nutritious?
- Consider your investments and the way you spend. Look after the pennies and the pounds will look after themselves.
- Consider your argument. Does it come from a place of fact and an attitude of wanting to sort things out, or a place of anger and intention to harm?
- Consider your home, is it a place of calm and sanctuary, what can you bring in or eliminate to reach this goal?
- Consider your neighbours, do you know them and are you building a community with them? It all begins with a simple "Hello".
- Consider your boss, or employees, are you making them feel valued and respected?
- Consider what you are wearing, is it appropriate? Will I be comfortable or am I just dressing to 'impress'?
- Consider the way you drive, and especially the way you park.
- Consider your tone of voice and attitude, when speaking to *anyone*, and *especially* to yourself.

Consider what you can do or say to be a blessing in someone's life today.

Thank you for reading this book. Please remember that etiquette is less about the 'doing to be *seen* to be doing', and more about doing something because you know it's the *right thing to do*.

We may not all dine with kings and hold a place at court, but we all possess our own little communities, these are *our* kingdoms. Your values, decency and small acts of kindness *will* raise those mighty nations.

If you want to change the world, go home and love your family.
Mother Teresa